KINGDOM MEN

RISE, LEAD, FINISH

Discover Your Identity
Gain Vision, and
Fulfill your Calling

Dusty Lapp

To every man who reads this book, I pray you see Jesus as He is…and become like Him.

KINGDOM MEN: RISE-LEAD-FINISH

Published by Dusty Lapp

Edited by Kristin Lapp

Cover and Interior Design and Layout by Dusty Lapp

Unless otherwise indicated, all scripture quotations are taken from the New King James Version of the Bible.

ISBN: 979-8-218-81631-5

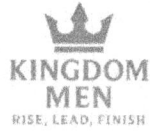

KINGDOM
MEN
RISE, LEAD, FINISH

KINGDOM MEN: RISE-LEAD-FINISH

Discover Your Identity,

Gain Vision, and

Fullfill Your Calling

DUSTY LAPP

CONTENTS

Foreword

Every generation faces a defining moment—a point in time when men must decide whether they will rise to the occasion or drift into complacency. We live in such a moment now. In a world where identity is confused, responsibility is avoided, and purpose is often lost in comfort, the need for Kingdom men has never been greater.

That's why this book is more than words on paper. It's a call to arms. Kingdom Men: Rise–Lead–Finish is a battle cry to every man who refuses to settle for mediocrity and longs to live with conviction, courage, and clarity.

Dusty Lapp writes with the authority of experience and the humility of a man who has fought his own battles. His journey—from the bull-fighting arena to ministry and mentorship—has forged in him a rare combination of grit and grace. What you'll find in these pages isn't theory. It's truth proven under pressure, wisdom gained through wounds, and hope born from a life fully surrendered to Christ.

This book will challenge you. It will confront the excuses that have kept you from stepping into your God-given potential. It will call out the passivity that has numbed too many hearts. But it will also equip you—with vision, identity, and a strategy to finish well.

The message of Kingdom Men is simple yet profound: transformation begins when a man aligns his spirit, soul, and body under the Lordship of Jesus Christ. From that place of unity flows power—power to lead your family, serve your community, and influence generations.

If you'll open your heart, this book will not just inform you; it will transform you. You'll find yourself rising with renewed strength, leading with divine purpose, and finishing the race with honor.

The Kingdom needs men who will rise. Men who will lead. Men who will finish. My prayer is that, as you turn these pages, you'll join the movement.

David J. Graham, D.Min
Founder and Lead Pastor of Kingdom Church,
Twin Falls, Idaho

PROLOGUE

This book is an honest look at the health of your spirit, soul, and body. If you're willing to look inward, it will challenge your core beliefs, confront your fears and doubts, require tough decisions—and ultimately help you grow into the image of Christ. That kind of transformation is essential if the Kingdom of God is going to expand in you and through you.

Many natural choices in life carry spiritual consequences. The health of your body, soul, and spirit creates ripple effects in your relationships, finances, and emotional life. Life is meant to be lived fully. But far too often, a lack of health in five key areas—spiritual, physical, relational, financial, and emotional—prevents people from stepping into their full potential. It isolates them from the life they were created to enjoy.

To get the most out of this book, you'll need commitment, vulnerability, tenacity, and courage. You must be willing to believe that God wants you whole—spirit, soul, and body—so you can partner with Holy Spirit to establish His Kingdom in your life and in the lives of those around you.

Here's what you'll discover: what you believe about yourself will shape your life more than what God believes about you. That's why my goal is to help you align your beliefs with what God says is true. My hope is that you become united in your being and your doing. Because unity is key.

Too many people walk through life with internal disunity. You desire health—but your choices don't agree with God's desires for you. When your soul (your mind, will, and emotions), your words, your intentions, and your actions all align, you become powerful. Not just for your own sake—but for the Kingdom's purpose. This power isn't aimless. It's not for self-help. It's the kind of power that sets you free so you can help bring heaven to earth—starting with your own life.

CHAPTER 1: The Power of Vision

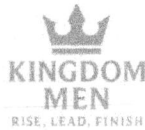

KINGDOM
MEN
RISE, LEAD, FINISH

Key Verse to memorize: "Where there is no vision, the people perish." — Proverbs 29:18 KJV

Vision brings focus, discipline, and direction. Without it, men drift. With it, men lead — and others follow.

Growing up in southern Idaho, I hunted with my dad in the high desert where sagebrush stretched as far as the eye could see. I remember asking him, "Where are we going?" Every time, his answer was the same: "Just over that hill." I already knew the answer—but I needed direction. From the backseat of his truck, the terrain looked endless. My small perspective couldn't grasp the vision he carried. I didn't know it then, but he wasn't aimlessly wandering. He had a destination in mind.

Most men today live like I did in that truck—staring at a wide open life, unsure where they're headed. Responsibilities pile up like endless hills, but without vision, purpose feels distant. Life becomes a barrage of distractions and you start reacting instead of leading. If you continue living like this, you will wake up years later and realize you've wandered far from who God called you to be.

A man without vision loses traction. He spins his wheels, burns fuel, and eventually breaks down never realizing his purpose.

Without vision, a man drifts. He loses his edge, his direction, and ultimately his identity. This causes him to forfeit his potential. But vision restores order. It calls you up. It breaks passivity.

This chapter isn't about dreaming—it's about *declaring the future God is building through you.*

Vision isn't about hype or ego—it's about clarity, conviction, and obedience. It's not about what you imagine, but what you inherit from God's heart. As a Kingdom man, your vision must come from God, not from culture or comparison. This chapter is a call to sharpen your spiritual eyes, to get clear on what God is building in you and through you.

Vision changes everything. Proverbs 29:18 says, "where there is no vision, the people perish" (KJV). Other translations read, 'people "cast off restraint.' Without a clear picture of where you're going, discipline fades and direction disappears, you lose the motivation to discipline your thoughts, habits, and decisions.

A man with vision is dangerous—in the best way. He becomes focused, grounded, and forward-moving. He is not reckless, but relentlessly locked onto vision.

Vision isn't just something you see—it's something you *fight* for. It is the divine picture of your future, given by God, that aligns your priorities, motivates your sacrifice, and is your God-given roadmap for your legacy.

Men today are starving for vision. We chase success, stimulation, and approval, but few are aware of (let alone focus on) vision. We know how to hustle, but not how to hear. We know how to grind, but not how to guard the purpose. We react instead of lead. Without vision, we default to distraction and distraction always leads to destruction.

When a man lacks vision, he becomes a slave to his surroundings. He surrenders his convictions to comfort. He trades his purpose for passivity. When vision fades, values collapse — and when values collapse, the man follows. But when a man *gains* vision—God-given, Kingdom-centered vision—he becomes dangerous to darkness and unstoppable in his mission.

Solution: God-Centered Vision

God has a vision for your health, your leadership, your family, your influence. And it's not vague or distant. Romans 12:2 says His will is "good, acceptable, and perfect." *Good*—there is nothing bad about His will for your life. *Acceptable*— you can receive what He has for you.

Perfect—it lacks nothing, it is complete. That's true not only for your spirit, but for your body, mind, and soul. He doesn't just want you to go to heaven. He wants His kingdom expressed through you—here and now. God's vision for your life is not vague or mystical—it's practical, purposeful, and personal. But to walk in that, you must want what God wants for you and see what God sees.

Jesus asked a blind man in **Mark 10:51**, "What do you want Me to do for you?" Jesus knew the man was blind, knew the man wanted his sight, yet still asked the question. The man knew Jesus had been the answer for so many others. Jesus wanted the blind man to know that He was the answer for him. Jesus wanted the man to see clearly, not fuzzy, not distorted, but clear. And, He wanted the blind man to be clear on what he wanted. Jesus didn't ask because He lacked knowledge—He asked to awaken desire.

Jesus still asks the same question today. "What do you want your life to look like?" Do you want what Jesus wants for you, or will you settle for what the world wants for you?

What do you want your spiritual, physical, relational, financial and emotional health to look like?

Do you know what you want your life to look like, or are you living by default? Until you answer that, you'll survive instead of lead.

Matthew 6:22-23 says, "The lamp of the body is the eye. If therefore your eye is good, your whole body will be full of light. But if your eye is bad, your whole body will be full of darkness. If therefore the light that is in you is darkness, how great is that darkness!" As we gain God's vision, His kingdom permeates every aspect of our lives. If we lack vision or have poor vision, darkness creeps into every aspect of our being. Your vision determines your direction and your direction determines your destiny.

Three Kinds of Vision

Foolish Vision – Proverbs 17:24 says, "…the eyes of a fool are on the ends of the earth." He has scattered goals, fragmented energy, and no direction.
- This man chases everything but builds nothing.

Problem-Centered Vision – This man has focus—but it's on the wrong thing. He obsesses over what's wrong instead of what could be right.
- This man magnifies what's broken but never believes it can be rebuilt.

God-Centered Vision – This man fixes his eyes on what God sees. He listens for the Father's voice, seeks the King's wisdom.
- This man aligns his life with heaven's blueprint.

MODERN DISTORTIONS

In the 1900s, families spent 43% of their income on food. By 2003, it dropped to 13%. We used to invest in our health because we had vision for life. Today, most men spend more on entertainment that numbs their souls rather than investing that money in ways that honor God with their spirit, soul and body. We feed cravings, not calling.

Disordered spending (of time and money) reveals disordered vision.

Your habits reveal your hope. Your spending reveals your story. If you looked at your time, your calendar, and your credit card statement, what would it say you value? What do they reveal concerning your spiritual, physical, relational, financial and emotional health?

Application: Living with Vision-Masculine Truth

A man without vision is a danger to himself and a liability to others. When you don't know your direction, you default to distraction, addiction, and passivity. But a man of vision walks in restraint, with discipline and conviction.

I am currently in my late 40's and I am passionately pursuing spiritual, physical, relational, financial and emotional health because my family deserves me at my best—so I can give them my best and lead them to theirs. If I'm not healthy; spirit, soul, and body, I can't lead my family into what God has for them. That is what compels me to fight for health. My "why" gives meaning to the pain of progress.

Biblical Anchor

Think of Nehemiah—he didn't just see broken walls; he envisioned a restored city. His vision fueled his courage, rallied men, and overcame opposition to finish the work. He had vision. And it made him effective. **Nehemiah 2:17-18**.

Coach's Corner

Every man must have a reason to fight through pain. Without one, the fight will break you. With one, the pain becomes preparation. Your vision fuels discipline. Vision defines direction. Vision gives purpose to your pain. Vision is prophetic. It sees what could be and chooses to live accordingly.

Vision must be

- *God-given* (not copied from culture)
- *Personal* (not generic)
- *Written* (not just thought about)
- *Guarded* (not easily swayed)

Core Ideas

- Vision gives purpose to your pain.
- Vision is prophetic. It sees what could be and chooses to live accordingly.
- Visionless men waste time, money, and energy.
- God gives vision, but you have to take responsibility to write it, live it, and protect it.

QUESTIONS

- What picture of my future is compelling enough to change my present?
- Where am I drifting (Spiritually, Physically, Relationally, Financially, and Emotionally) because I lack vision?
- What would be different if I wasn't drifting in these areas?
- What desires has God put in my heart that I've been ignoring?

- Does my calendar match my calling?
- Am I living out someone else's expectations—or God's vision for my life?

Action

Take 20 minutes today. Sit in silence. Ask Holy Spirit: "What is Your vision for my life, in these 5 areas: (Spiritual, Physical, Emotional, Relational, Financial), and what do I need to do or know to increase my health and leadership in them?"

Write what you hear. Then, write a one-paragraph **Vision Statement** that starts with, "I exist to...," Or, "My life will..."

Example: "I exist to lead my family into the presence and purpose of God every day."

If it's fuzzy at first, keep coming back. The more you ask, the clearer it becomes. Keep it simple. Don't worry about getting it "right"—just start.

On a scale of 1-10, rate your level of health in all 5 areas (Spiritual, physical, relational, financial, emotional). Ask Holy Spirit what it will take to increase that number in each area.

Challenge

Memorize Proverbs 29:18. Speak it out every morning this week before you step into your day.

For the next 7 days, speak your vision out loud every morning. Tape it to your bathroom mirror.

Remind your soul: "This is who I am. This is where I'm going. This is what God has for me."

Journal Prompt

- Where have I been living without vision?
- What has it cost me?
- What needs to change so I can gain vision and stay focused on it?
- What will change if I start today?

Closing Thoughts

Vision isn't something you stumble into—it's something you seek, fight for, and protect. Without it, you drift. With it, you advance—actively participating in God's Kingdom being established here on earth as it is in Heaven. Now's the time.

Get clear. Get focused. Get after it.

Chapter 2: Shoulder Your Responsibility as a Man

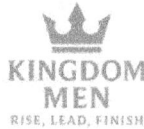

KINGDOM
MEN
RISE, LEAD, FINISH

Key Verses to memorize: *"When I was a child, I spoke as a child, I thought as a child: but when I became a man, I put away childish things."* — **1 Corinthians 13:11**

"Maturity doesn't come with age, but with the acceptance of responsibility." – *Dr. Edwin Louis* Cole

Real men don't make excuses—they take responsibility. Maturity isn't automatic; it's intentional it doesn't come with age, it comes with the acceptance of Responsibility. Responsibility is not a burden—it's a mantle. It's the mark of Kingdom manhood. This chapter is about breaking the back of passivity and embracing the authority and responsibility God gave you to lead. No one else is coming. You are the man for the job.

Problem: Abdication and Passivity- Hung Up

I used to teach bullfighting at Lyle Sankey's rodeo schools. One of the most important lessons I'd teach the riders was about what to do if they got hung up—when you're riding hand binds in the rope and you can't get free from the bull. I'd walk them through what the bullfighters would do to work the hang up, and what they needed to do-first thing being, open their hand. Then I'd ask: **"If you get hung up, whose responsibility** is it to get your hand out?"

One kid said, "It's the bullfighter's job to get us out."
I looked him square in the face and asked,
"Did the bullfighter pay your entry fee?"
"Did he put your hand in your rope?"
"Did he make you nod your head?"

No. **You did.**

It's your rope. Your ride. Your responsibility. If you get hung, its on you. You need to get your hand out. Situations and circumstances will continue to drag you around and beat you up as long as you continue waiting for someone else to help you.

The same goes for life: Don't hang and drag and wait to be rescued. Open your hand! Let go of old ways of thinking, habits and relationships that are destroying your spiritual, physical, financial, relational and emotional health...**Fight to get free.**

Nobody forced you to make the decisions you've made, or ignore red flags. You may have faced pain, trauma, or disadvantage—but at some point, you must **own your response**. STOP dragging and start leading.

Most men don't fall into poor health out of ignorance. They fall into it through passivity, avoidance, and because they never took ownership.

Stop blaming others. Stop waiting to be rescued. Start taking responsibility.

God's Word on Responsibility

In Genesis 1:26–28, God gave mankind dominion. That means **leadership, stewardship, ownership, responsibility**. He gave Adam a garden to tend, protect, and cultivate. But when things went wrong, Adam blamed Eve,—then God, and then tried to hide from God.

When God calls out to Adam, "Where are you?" He is not asking for Himself, He is asking so Adam can own his actions and acknowledge that he shrugged off the responsibility God has entrusted to him. Adam was handed responsibility, he handed it off, and needed to own it. This same story still plays out today. God entrusts men with responsibility. We either **lead it or lose it**.

God asks us the same questions: **"Where are you, man?"** (Genesis 3:9)

He's not looking for someone to blame. He's looking for someone to take responsibility. Until you know where you are, you can't get where God wants you to go.

Solution: Rejecting Passivity Embrace Responsibility

We live in a culture that glorifies blame, immaturity, and victimhood. It promotes passivity as if it's noble. But Kingdom men take ownership. Kingdom men **reject cultural agreements** and shoulder the responsibility of what God has entrusted to them.

When we agree with culture, we align with the enemy and tolerate what will eventually destroy us. Not much has changed since Adam. American culture has been increasingly bent toward the idea that husbands and wives are to "submit to one another." Churches quote Ephesians 5:21 in support of this idea, not understanding that the submission in verse 21 is referring to submitting to other members of the body of Christ. Verses 22-24 specifies the wife is to submit to her own husband and is not under the authority of other men. Understanding this authority structure, and living in it, opens up the Kingdom of Heaven in our lives. When we abdicate our responsibility and go against this structure by being passive, we leave a door open for the enemy to come in and fill that leadership position.

Every man has unknowingly made agreements with the kingdom of darkness. Every agreement gives the enemy legal access. But repentance breaks that access—and **responsibility begins the process of restoration**.

If you shake hands with worldly culture, you are coming into agreement with the enemy. You are aligning your life with what the enemy says rather than what God says, and in so doing, you are giving the enemy legal access to invade your life. If this is you…and make no mistake, it is, only repentance can break the legal authority you have handed to the enemy. Every man has made agreements with the enemy and allowed the kingdom of darkness to have legal access to areas of their lives. The question is, how long will you tolerate the enemy? How long will you settle for a truce rather than a victory?

This is your wake-up call. You were made to lead—not because you're flawless, but because God works through responsible men to deliver Kingdom answers (Ezekiel 22:30). His Kingdom is the answer to any and all issues the world faces. He repeatedly shows us that He uses men to bring those answers… A Kingdom man is different. He doesn't shift blame. He doesn't abdicate. He doesn't wait for rescue. He stands up and takes ownership of what God has entrusted to him. Consider David when he killed Uriah. When confronted, David took responsibility and repented. God isn't focused on the sin, His focus is on restoring us from sin. That restoration comes only after we take responsibility and repent.

Physical Health:

God didn't give you a body so you could outsource its care to a doctor or hope insurance would fix it when it breaks. He gave it to you so you could rule over it. And ruling it means owning it. Everything you put in your body matters. Healthy food = healthy body. Garbage food = sickness and disease.

Stop Abdicating your physical health. Start Leading.

We've created a culture where men abdicate responsibility and then blame the results on God. I see too many men saying things like, "If God wanted me healthy, He'd heal me." The truth is, God wants you healthy, and He wants you to be a man who takes responsibility for his choices.

Stop choosing food that harms your body. To continue eating junk and praying for God to heal you is tempting God. You may say, "I'm just trusting the Lord to work it all out." Yes—trust God. But saying you are trusting God and then ignoring your responsibility is not trust at all. It's immaturity and an excuse to be lazy.

There's a lie that your physical health doesn't have a spiritual impact. But Scripture says otherwise:

- You were created in the image of God (Genesis 1:27).
- Jesus died to redeem and heal both soul and body (Isaiah 53:5).
- Your body is the temple of the Holy Spirit (1 Corinthians 6:19)
- Your body matters and you must take responsibility for your physical health.

Your health is your responsibility.

Don't abdicate what God called you to steward. Faith without works is dead (James 2:17). Faith is proven through your action.

Responsibility is the **action of faith**. This action needs to be applied to your Spiritual, Financial, Relational, and Emotional health, just like it does to your physical health. Stop waiting for someone to come rescue you.

Application: Living as a Responsible Man Masculine Focus:

- Responsibility is not a burden—it's a mantle. When you stop waiting to be rescued and start owning your role, you become dangerous to darkness and an asset in the Kingdom of heaven.
- Maturity doesn't come with age, but with the acceptance of responsibility and is the road a man walks that leads to transformation.
- Victimhood is easy. **Ownership is transformation.**
- Kingdom men don't make excuses—they make Kingdom minded decisions.
- A responsible man is **dangerous to darkness**. Kingdom men don't blame, **they build.**

Coach's Corner

Every area you avoid will eventually collapse. But every area you take responsibility for, God can build His Kingdom in you.

You can't lead others if you won't lead yourself.

When you stop waiting to be rescued and start owning your role, **you become an asset in God's Kingdom.**

Core Ideas

- Reject the temptation to abdicate responsibility.
- You are responsible for your spiritual, physical, relational, financial and emotional health.
- Every area you avoid will eventually collapse.
- Maturity, authority, and influence all begin with **acceptance of responsibility**.
- Accepting responsibility is what activates Kingdom impact.

Questions

- Where have I blamed others instead of owning my part?
- How has this stopped me from discovering God's vision for me?
- What lies have I believed about my ability to change?
- Where have I passively waited to be rescued instead of answering God's call for me to lead with courage?
- Where is God calling me to stop excusing and start executing?
- What will my life look like in 1 year if I keep living how I am right now?
- How would my life change if I took full responsibility today?
- Where am I tolerating immaturity or making excuses?
- Am I stewarding or squandering my spiritual, physical, relational, financial and emotional health?

Journal Prompts

- What does manhood look like when I own every decision, outcome, and opportunity God has placed in my hands?
- What areas of life have I been waiting for someone else to rescue me?
- Where have I been living like a boy instead of a man?

- What have I been tolerating, excusing, or postponing?
- What will shift in my life when I take full responsibility?

Action

Write this statement and say it aloud every morning:
"I take full responsibility for my spiritual, physical, relational, financial, and emotional health. I refuse to blame. God gave me dominion, and I will steward it well."

Identify one area you've neglected or blamed others for. Then take one bold step this week—no matter how small, to lead in that area.

Make it simple. Make it doable. **Own it.**

Closing Thought

Maturity doesn't happen by accident. It begins the moment a man says:**"No one else is coming. I've got this. God gave it to me, He trust me and will lead me. I will steward it well."**

You can't always control what happens to you. But you can always control your response. And response is the foundation of responsibility.

Stop making excuses. Start making progress.

Chapter 3: Identity in Christ

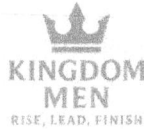

KINGDOM
MEN
RISE, LEAD, FINISH

Key Verses to memorize:
"The Spirit Himself bears witness with our spirit that we are God's children." — *Romans 8:16*

"You have put on the new man, who is renewed in knowledge according to the image of Him who created him.
— *Colossians 3:10*

"Then God said, 'Let Us make man in Our image, according to Our likeness...' — *Genesis 1:26*

"For as many as are led by the Spirit of God, these are the sons of God." —**Romans 8:14**

"For the earnest expectation of the creation eagerly waits for the revealing of the sons of God."— **Romans 8:19**

Identity Matters:

What image do you portray? Our friends, our clothes, our tattoos (or lack thereof), coffee shops or bar stools, we look to all of these things and more to prop up an image that we take as our own....an image for ourselves created by ourselves. What would the world look like if our desire was to be shaped into His image...to take on His image...to become like Him? It is good to stop striving, stop trying to measure up, stop trying to look the part, just allow His image and character to be formed in you. This is where peace is found. Let Him shape you. You are found in Him. He created you "To become like Him," **Genesis 1:26**

You can't walk in authority until you know who you are. A man unsure of his identity will either drift aimlessly or fight battles that aren't his. Until you know your identity in Christ, you'll live like someone you're not—defined by your past success and failure, past wounds, false labels, and cultural expectations. But when you discover who you are as a son of God, everything changes.

You weren't created to live like an orphan. You are a son of the Most High God. Your true identity doesn't come from your job, your failures, or your family history—it comes from your Father. This chapter is a call to war against false labels and reclaim your God-given identity. Your name, your nature, and your mission come from your Father—not from your past, your pain, or your paycheck.

Every man is living from an identity—either one the world gave him, or one his past shaped, or the one his Father in heaven declared. Until you know who you are in Christ, you'll keep trying to prove, perform, and pretend. But when you walk in sonship, everything changes.

If you don't know who you are, someone else will decide for you.

- Culture will label you.

- Failure will define you.

- Your past will haunt you.

- And insecurity will rule you.

But when you know your identity in Christ, you stop living for approval—and start living from it.

The Image You Carry

God created man in His image (**Genesis 1:26**). That means you were designed to reflect His strength, character, leadership, creativity, and integrity.

Sin distorted that image, but Jesus came not just to forgive sin—but to **restore your identity**.

You're not here to perform. You're here to reflect the King.

Problem: False Identities and Orphan Living

Many men live under false identities. At times, I've lived under all of them.

- **The Tough Guy** – Hides emotion. Never shows weakness.

- **The Doer** – Ties worth to income, title, or performance.

- **The People Pleaser** – Avoids conflict. Never leads.

- **The Prover** – Grinds endlessly. Always proving. Never enough.

But these are identities we **earn**—and what can be earned can be lost. In Christ, your identity isn't earned. **It's received. Only sonship is secure. You are a son.**

Solution: Receiving What God Says About You

If you are in Christ:

- You are a **new creation (2 Corinthians 5:17)**.

- You are **righteous and holy (Ephesians 4:24)**.

- You are a **son of God (Galatians 4:6–7)**.

- You are **forgiven and free (Romans 6:6–7)**.

- You are a **warrior with divine authority (Ephesians 6:10–18)**.

You don't have to fake it, earn it, or prove it. You just have to receive it and walk in it.

Masculine Focus

A man will never lead boldly until he believes deeply that he is who God says he is. When your identity is secure, you stop striving to prove yourself and start living to glorify God. When you root your confidence in Christ, you stop chasing validation and start walking in purpose.

- Insecurity is the byproduct of misplaced identity.

- Sons walk with confidence. Orphans walk in fear and insecurity.

- Too many grown men are still living like spiritual orphans—striving, hiding, comparing, and never feeling "enough."

You are a son of the most High God. Walk like it.

The Name I Answer To

Gideon was hiding in fear when the angel of the Lord called him, "Mighty man of valor!"— Judges 6:11. At that moment, Gideon didn't feel mighty—but God was calling Gideon who he was, not who Gideon thought he was. He was calling out who Gideon was meant to be. Who he needed to be, and who the people around him needed him to be. If he didn't step into who God called him to be, people around him would remain oppressed and in bondage. This is true for you as well. If you fail to own your identity as a son of God, people around you will suffer the consequences.

Identity isn't about how you feel—it's about what God declares.

You've heard the saying, "fake it till you make it." The sentiment means well, but it's garbage thinking. As sons of God we don't "fake it till we make it"—we **believe it because He said it**.
You are already who God says you are—you just need to walk in it.

The same was true for David, Joseph, Peter, and even Jesus. Each faced an identity test **before** stepping into their assignment.

Training horses was a part of my past. Horses, as prey animals, are driven by fear and survival instincts, including eating, sleeping, and breeding. However, horses have immense potential that can be unleashed through training and goes beyond what they could ever do alone.

A horse's first instinct is to scatter when it's afraid. It thinks that escape is safer than facing the trainer. This reaction comes from fear and past experiences. Yet, with consistent guidance and patience, horses discover that their true safety, and the ability to unlock their incredible capacity, such as working with cattle, lies in submitting to the trainer's direction. When it submits to the trainer, it goes from just a horse to a horse that is useful.

Men are no different. Freedom has been given, along with a new identity. But without actively submitting to Him by renewing our mind to who He is and who He says we are, it is impossible to fully grasp and live out the potential God has put in us from birth. (**Ephesians 2:10**).

We have been set free. We've been given identity. But if we don't renew our mind, we'll continue to live driven by fear and self preservation.

Application: Walk in Identity
The War Between Old and New

Romans 7 paints a picture of two identities at war:

- The **Old Man** – Driven by shame, fear, and self-preservation.— **Ephesians 4:22**

- The **New Man** – Empowered by the Spirit to walk in freedom.— **Ephesians 4:24**

The battleground is your soul—your thoughts, emotions, and decisions. If your soul hasn't been renewed by His Spirit, you'll live divided. You'll **want** to live in truth but keep falling back into lies.

That's why identity must move from **head to heart**, from **theology to reality,** from **belief to** behavior.

You don't fight for identity. You fight **from** identity.

Coach's Corner

- Every attack on your life is an attack on your identity. The enemy fears a man who knows who he is.

- Jesus didn't start His ministry until the Father said, "This is My Son, in whom I am well pleased." Identity came before assignment.

- You weren't made to hustle for your worth. You were made to carry your Father's name and commanded "do not take the name of the Lord your God in vain." You have been given His name, which holds His power and authority. You have responsibility for that. If you live like like that is not a reality, you have taken His name in vain.

Core Ideas

- You are not what you do. You are not what others did to you.

- You are who God says you are: **chosen, loved, equipped, called**.

- Identity leads to integrity. Knowing who you are leads to living the life Jesus came to give.

- You can't live a new life while believing old lies.

Questions

- What names or labels have I been living under that God never gave me?

- What lies have shaped my story that need to be broken today?

- How has my past shaped my identity more than my Father?

- Am I trying to earn love—or, am I living from it?

- Where am I performing instead of resting in who God says I am?

- What would change if I truly believed I was a son of God?

Action Step

Write your **identity declaration** using this format:
"Because I am in Christ, I am His son. I no longer identify with ____.
I receive what God says about me, and I will walk in it today."

Fill in the blanks. Be honest. Make it your own. Then speak it aloud every morning this week.

Challenge

Write down the top 3 lies you've believed about yourself (e.g., "I'm not enough," "I always fail," "I'm too far gone").

Then find and write out 3 Scriptures that speak truth to each lie. Tape them where you'll see them daily. Declare them over your life and let your mind be renewed. (If you don't know how to find 3 verses- ask a brother for help).

Stand in front of a mirror this week and declare: **"I am a son of God. I am chosen. I am loved. I am not who I was—I am who God says I am."**

Repeat it until your heart believes what your mouth is saying.

Journal Prompt

Ask Holy Spirit:

- What lie about my identity has held me back the most?

- What truth do I need to believe instead?

- What would my life look like if I walked daily in my true identity?

Closing Thought

A man of God doesn't find his identity in what he's done. He finds it in what Christ has done **for him**. You don't need to prove yourself you need to be who God says you are.

When you know who you are, you stop chasing the approval of the world and start advancing the Kingdom with boldness, clarity, and confidence.

You weren't made to hustle for your worth.

Live like a son. Carry your Father's name. And walk in the authority that comes from identity.

Chapter 4: What You Consume

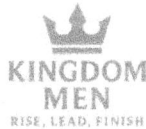

KINGDOM
MEN
RISE, LEAD, FINISH

Key Verses to Memorize:

"whether you eat or drink, or whatever you do, do all to the glory of God." — *1* **Corinthians 10:31**

"All things are lawful for me, but not all things are helpful... I will not be brought under the power of anything." — **1 Corinthians 6:12** (ASV)

"No discipline seems pleasant at the time, but painful. Later on, however, it produces a harvest of righteousness and peace for those who have been trained by it." — *Hebrews 12:11* (NIV)

Jesus is the Bread of Life

In **John 6:35, 48**, and **51** Jesus tells us that He is "the bread of life." When He is teaching us how to pray in **Matthew 6:5-15** he tells us we are to ask God to "give us this day our daily bread."

The way a man eats reveals more than just his physical health—it reveals discipline, mindset, purpose, priorities, stewardship, and his relationship with control. If we want to change our health, we must first change our thinking. This chapter confronts the deeper motivations behind our food choices. Please don't think too narrowly when I say "food choices." Expand your thinking to include, not only food for your body, but the daily bread we need from God in order to establish His kingdom in us and around us. We are shaped by what our body, soul, and spirit consume daily.

God tells us that He prepares a table before us in the presence of our enemies (**Psalm 23:5**). Jesus declares that He is the bread of life and instructs us to ask the Father for our daily bread. He also reminds Satan that man does not live by bread alone, but by every word that proceeds from the mouth of God (**Matthew 4:4**).

In these statements, Jesus takes something physical and natural—bread—and connects it to a spiritual truth that impacts every area of our lives.

Now consider this: we sit at many tables in life. At each one, we have the opportunity to consume what God offers—or what the world offers. We can sit at the table of a fast-food restaurant and eat highly processed food, or we can sit at the dinner table and enjoy quality, properly prepared, nutrient-dense, whole food.

The table we choose directly impacts our health—physically and spiritually.

So ask yourself:

• Which tables do you find yourself frequenting?

- Are you fueling your mission or feeding your emotions?

- Are you fueling your mission or numbing the pain?

- Are you disciplining your body or destroying it?

Kingdom men lead at the table.

Distracted and Dependent

We live in a world of processed convenience. We grab what's easy. We snack between meetings. We reward ourselves with sugar and caffeine like we're children.

Then we pray for health, while still bowing to cravings.

It's time to grow up. As men of God, we must learn to **steward** our plates—not be slaves to them.

When Jesus was tempted in the wilderness after fasting, Satan attacked His identity through food: "If You are the Son of God, turn these stones into bread."

The battle wasn't just about bread—it was about **identity**.

A man who can't say no to food will struggle to say yes to God.

I've worked with men who could deadlift 400 lbs—but couldn't say no to a sleeve of Oreos. I've seen pastors preach sermons on discipleship and self discipline—then gorge themselves at the church potluck. I knew a friend who laughed off journaling his meals—until he did it for three days. "I didn't realize how much I was stress eating until I saw it written down" he said.

These aren't weak men. They're just unaware that their food choices are often **emotional and spiritual decisions wearing physical disguises.**

The Hidden Drivers Behind Your Food Choices

Most men don't actually have a food problem—they have a focus problem. We often eat for reasons that have nothing to do with real hunger:

- **Stress** – Food becomes an escape after a hard day.

- **Control** – Life feels chaotic, but the plate feels controllable.

- **Boredom** – Restlessness disguises itself as hunger.

- **Emotion** – Sadness, anger, anxiety, or loneliness trigger a food fix.

- **Identity**" – This is just how I've always eaten."

The truth is, we eat in alignment with the beliefs we carry about ourselves. If you believe you're undisciplined or broken, your food choices will reflect that. You won't eat like a King's son while still thinking like a slave.

The Deeper Problem

The world has taught us to see food as more than fuel. Because of this, food often reveals what's really going on inside us:

- **Comfort** – Food exposes our source of comfort. Too many men use it to replace Holy Spirit—the One who is meant to be our true Comforter.

- **Control** – Food reveals who's really in charge. Are we controlled by our flesh, or led by the Spirit?

- **Culture** – Food reflects the culture we accept. Too often, men go along with unhealthy cultural norms instead of establishing Kingdom culture in their homes and communities.

- **Distraction** – Food can act as an escape. Distractions scratch an itch that keeps us pacified while deeper problems fester. The answer isn't numbing ourselves—it's removing distractions, facing the problem, and asking Holy Spirit to heal us.

- **Reward** – Food becomes a way to satisfy the flesh, but it leaves us spiritually soft and undisciplined.

That's why the real question isn't just *what* you eat—but *why* you eat it.

Are you fueling the mission—or feeding your emotions?

Are you eating to live—or living to eat?

Kingdom Principle

Kingdom men don't see food as a substitute savior—they see it as fuel for their assignment. Every meal is an opportunity to either strengthen the body to carry out God's purpose or weaken it by bowing to the flesh. The choice is never just about calories or cravings—it's about whether you're aligning with your identity as a son of the King or settling for the chains of slavery.

33

God wants you healthy—spirit, soul, and body. Our Greek mindset works best when everything is tucked neatly into separate compartments. That can be helpful at times, but it also blinds us to the bigger picture of how everything is connected. One mindset that has crept into the church— and stifled God's Kingdom from being fully established on earth—is the belief that the physical isn't as important as the spiritual.

This thinking runs so deep that many people will nod in agreement when they hear it, as if analyzing two separate realities, without realizing the glaring truth: the physical *is* spiritual. They are one.

Oneness is hard for us to grasp because we love to compartmentalize. Yet God desires us to be one, just as He is One. We often miss how something as simple as a poor diet of processed food can have a destructive ripple effect on every part of life—spirit, soul, and body.

Think about it: going for a run or hitting the gym isn't just about burning calories—it's training your body to have the stamina to serve others when God calls. Choosing to eat whole, life-giving foods isn't just "nutrition"—it's stewardship, an act of worship that honors the temple of the Holy Spirit. Even something as basic as sleep becomes a spiritual discipline when you see how rest sharpens your mind, strengthens your emotions, and fuels your ability to hear God's voice.

Spiritually, people are dying before they ever fulfill what God has placed in their hearts to accomplish. What a disservice to a lost and dying world. What if *you* are the answer your neighbor needs, but your health keeps you from showing up—whether to share God's love or lend a helping hand in their time of need?

That picture may be about as subtle as a bee down the pants—but sometimes we need a wake-up call that sharp.

Some men are sick in their bodies because their souls are not healthy.

3 John 1:2 says, *"Beloved, I pray that you may prosper in all things and be in health, just as your soul prospers."* In other words, the health of your soul influences the health of your body—and even your prosperity in life.

Too often, when people hear the word "prosperity," they immediately think about money. They put themselves in a box. But the freedom Christ came to give us blows the walls off that box.

Prosperity isn't just financial—it's for *every area of life.* To limit it to money is actually a sign of an unhealthy soul, because it shuts you off from the fullness of God's prosperity in your relationships, health, purpose, emotions, and every other area of life.

Your soul—your mind, will, and emotions—is the hinge point of health. When your soul prospers, your health prospers. But if your soul is unhealthy, your body will eventually show it.

Think about it:

- Is a prosperous **mind** full of thoughts that contradict God's Word? Or is it renewed and anchored in truth?

- Is a prosperous **will** rigid and stubborn because of pride? Or is it surrendered, flexible, and aligned with the Holy Spirit?

- Are your **emotions** prospering—or are they consumed with anger, jealousy, bitterness, and unforgiveness?

If you want your body to prosper, these soul issues have to be addressed.

The way you think can literally create health problems. A will that refuses to yield to God breeds stress and exhaustion. If you believe you're the creator and sustainer of your world, you carry a crushing weight you were never designed to bear—a load that will eventually break your body.

And emotions? They are directly tied to your physical condition. Stress, anxiety, fear, anger, bitterness, hatred, discouragement—all of these poison your body from the inside out.

Within the soul, the **mind is the captain.** It gives direction to the will and the emotions. The mind brings order to the team. But when your mind is undisciplined, your emotions spin out of control, and your will becomes either weak and breakable or hard and prideful—both equally destructive.

That's why Scripture tells us to *"be transformed by the renewing of your mind"* (**Romans 12:2**). The mind is the battlefield where health is won or lost.

Think of it like a tree. Your body is the fruit, but your soul is the root system. If the roots are rotting—filled with bitterness, fear, or pride—the fruit will always be sickly. But if the roots are healthy—anchored in Jesus, yielded to His will, and alive with His Spirit—then the fruit will be strong, nourishing, and full of life. A prosperous soul produces a prosperous body.

Solution: Stewardship and Submission God Cares About What You Eat—

Here's Why

It's not about legalism—it's about **lordship**.

1 Corinthians 10:31 reminds us to eat and drink for the glory of God. That means even what you put on your plate is part of your purpose.

Your food choices affect:

- Your clarity of thought.

- Your ability to lead under pressure.

- Your emotional resilience.

- Your energy for work, family, and ministry.

- Your recovery, sleep, and long-term vitality.

A man ruled by his appetite cannot be trusted with spiritual authority. But a man who rules his appetite can lead nations (**See Daniel chapter 1**).

It would be remiss to look past the examples in the Old Testament where God commanded sacrifices to restore what had been broken. If we look deeper, we can see all of these sacrifices were food. They were something that could be consumed that God asked to be sacrificed.

Food as a Spiritual Issue

Most men compartmentalize life: "*This* is spiritual. *This* is physical. *This* is just food."

But in the Kingdom, **nothing is compartmentalized**. Your body is not disconnected from your purpose.

If you're constantly foggy, inflamed, crashing from sugar, or living on stimulants—you are not at full capacity. And if you're not at full capacity, you can't carry the full weight of your calling.

Every bite either fuels your purpose—or feeds your flesh. Your body is a temple, if the table is your altar, is your worship acceptable to God?

Biblical Anchor: Daniel

Daniel "purposed in his heart" not to defile himself with the king's food (**Daniel 1:8**). His appetite was aligned with his assignment.

Daniel's decision to steward his body didn't make him weaker—it made him **sharper, stronger, and more favored.**

Daniel didn't just honor God with his mind or spirit—he honored Him with his diet.

Masculine Focus

- Food is fuel for your **mission**. It's preparation so you can lead, serve, protect, and build.

- It's not about six-packs or fad diets—it's about **strength for the calling**.

- You are either training for battle or surrendering to comfort.

- What you put in your mouth is either building your body or breaking it down.

- Your stomach is not just about satisfaction—it's about **submission**.

- Kingdom men lead themselves—even at the table.

Core Ideas

- Food for my soul, physical food, and spiritual food, are not neutral—what you consume impacts your ability to lead, serve, and endure.

- Most eating/consumption is emotional—identify the emotion and return to God's truth.

- God doesn't demand perfection, but He expects **stewardship** (**Matthew 25:14–30**).

- Stewarding your body reflects **spiritual maturity**.

Questions

- Why do I eat what I eat—hunger, habit, or healing?

- When I'm stressed, tired, or angry—do I reach for brownies or my Bible?

- Is what I am eating building me up—or breaking me down?

- Do my food habits reflect my Kingdom assignment or emotional cravings?

- What role does food play in my reward system, identity, or self-worth?

Challenge

Ask Holy Spirit what **trigger food or drink** He is asking you to remove.

- Sugary drinks, alcohol, sugar, bread, fast food, nightly snacks etc.

- Replace it with a nutrient-dense option.

Pay attention to what shifts—not just physically, but emotionally and spiritually as you begin feeding your mission instead of your emotions. It's important to identity this because you can't change what you won't confront.

Then ask Holy Spirit: **What am I really hungry for? Where am I needing you to heal me?**

Journal Prompts

- If I saw food for my spirit, soul, and body as fuel for God's purpose, how would it change what I consume?

- How has my relationship with food reflected my beliefs about God, myself, and my purpose?

- What needs to change—and what would change if I began to fuel my life with **intention instead of impulse?**

Closing Thought

God isn't trying to restrict your joy—He's trying to increase your strength. You can't fight the good fight while you are subject to your cravings.

A man ruled by his appetite will always remain a slave. But a man who rules his appetite can be trusted with authority.

Discipline your plate. Don't be a slave to it. Fuel the mission.

KINGDOM MEN

Chapter 5: Find Your "Why"

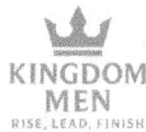

KINGDOM
MEN
RISE, LEAD, FINISH

Key Verses to Memorize

"For David, after he had served the purpose of God in his own generation, fell asleep..." — **Acts 13:36** (ESV)

"To everything there is a season, a time for every purpose under heaven."—**Ecclesiasties 3:1** (KJV)

"Looking unto Jesus, the author and finisher of our faith, who for the joy that was set before Him endured the cross, despising the shame, and has sat down at the right hand of the throne of God." — **Hebrews 12:2** (KJV)...*For the Joy set before Him*

"Counsel in the heart of man is like deep water, but a man of understanding will draw it out." — **Proverbs 20:5**

"Where there is no vision, the people perish." — **Proverbs 29:18** (KJV)

A man with a *why* can endure almost any *how*. Without purpose, men drift. They become passive, distracted, addicted, and disengaged. But when a man discovers his God-given why, he becomes focused, fueled, and formidable.

Discipline without direction always ends in burnout. Motivation fades, but purpose endures. If you want to finish the race, you need more than a plan—you need a purpose. Your *why* isn't a slogan or motivational quote; it's a Kingdom assignment. It's not about fame, comfort, or success. It's about knowing why you exist and living every day with that clarity.

This chapter challenges you to discover your *why*—and live like it matters.

The Problem: Motivation Isn't Enough

Our culture is obsessed with motivation—quotes, playlists, speeches, even pre-workout drinks. But motivation doesn't last. It's like an adrenaline rush: it feels great for a moment, but it always wears off, leaving you restless and searching for the next hit. They keep searching for an external push because they haven't tapped into their internal purpose.

Men who live by motivation quit when life gets hard. Men who live by purpose push through the pain.

Your *why* is what keeps you moving when:

- Your body says quit.

- The mountain seems too big.

- No one notices your effort.

Your *why* is the fuel that keeps you steady when everything else says stop. If you don't know why you do what you do, you won't last.

The Wake-Up Call

John Maxwell says, *"Value the process more than events."*

I remember a conversation with Mike (name changed for privacy). I think his exact words were "we are in a dog fight." His words were filled with emotion, urgency, and regret, all packaged up in a good gut punch. His wife had just been diagnosed with Hashimoto's disease. For years, sleepless nights, fatigue, and mood swings had been accepted as "normal"—until the diagnosis made it clear something was deeply wrong.

As we talked through family history, Mike shared that his wife's family was marked by diabetes and Alzheimer's. What shook him most was an incident of severe brain fog: his wife showed up for a doctor's appointment on the wrong day—in the wrong month.

Mike admitted that due to his wife's family history of Alzheimers, this incident "scared the crap" out of him. That moment brought his why into clarity. Love. Conviction. Purpose.

Mike realized that how he led his family, stocked the fridge, and stewarded their health would shape their future. Willpower hadn't been enough. But when he found his purpose, he found fresh energy to lead.

Solution: Why Purpose Beats Willpower

Willpower is like a battery. You wake up with a charge, but stress, temptation, and resistance drain it quickly. Willpower alone becomes self-reliance. If you're like me, you've been there and when you are there, you quickly realize, "white-knuckling" life will always leave you exhausted.

Purpose is different. Purpose speaks to identity. It doesn't fade—it fuels.

Stephen Covey put it this way: *"How different our lives are when we really know what is deeply important to us, and keeping that picture in mind, we manage ourselves each day to be and to know what matters most."*

When you understand the "Why" behind your purpose, it connects your habits to your mission:

* Not, "I want abs."

  But, *"I want to be the dad my kids want to follow."*

* Not, *"I want to lose weight."*

  But, *"I want to finish the race God marked out for me."*

Purpose helps us order our lives in a way that causes our thoughts, actions, intentions, and words to work together. When your purpose is clear, your discipline becomes powerful.

Masculine Truth

* You weren't made to just survive—you were made to lead, build, and leave a legacy.

* Your purpose isn't about ego or fame—it's about assignment. It's not about you. Your purpose is given to you for the benefit of others.

- A man with a purpose stops chasing pleasure and starts focusing his time, energy, resources, and intentions on that purpose. He builds with conviction.

- Your Purpose is your God-given reason for being alive in this generation. When you understand your "Why" behind this purpose, you are unstoppable.

Without a "why" your strength will fail. But understanding "why" your pain becomes preparation. Discover it. Then live like it matters, because it does.

Climbing the Wrong Mountain

John Maxwell once said, *"If we don't have a plan and purpose for our lives, we will become part of someone else's."*

Years ago I met a man who had climbed the ladder of business success—money, influence, status. But his health was wrecked, his family didn't know him and he had no peace.

Through tears, he talked with me about how he had climbed to the top of the mountain only to realized he had climbed the wrong mountain.

That's what happens when we pursue the world's definition of success instead of God's vision for our lives.

Biblical Anchor: David

Acts 13:36 says, *"David served the purpose of God in his own generation."*

David wasn't perfect. But he was purposeful. He fought giants, led kingdoms, repented with humility, and worshipped with abandon. Why? Because he knew his assignment.

Purpose doesn't require perfection. It requires surrender.

Core Ideas

- You were made on purpose—for a purpose.

- God gives desires not for comfort, but for His Kingdom.

- Your *purpose* needs to be the filter for your decisions.

- Without purpose men drift, perform, or people-please.

- Your why anchors you when life gets hard.

- Your purpose must be bigger than your pain.

Questions for Reflection

- What has God wired me to build, lead, protect, or restore?

- Where have I traded calling for comfort?

- What legacy do I want to leave—and what's keeping me from it?

- What battle burns in my heart that I can't ignore?

- What do I want my spiritual, physical, financial, relational, and emotional health to look like in 5 years? Why docs that matter?

- Who will suffer if I don't change? What will be different if I do?

- When I feel like quitting, what will remind me why I started?

Action: Drill Down Your Why

Use this simple exercise to find your why:

1. Start with: *"I want to be healthy because _____."*

2. Then ask: *"Why is that important?"*

3. Repeat 3–5 times, digging deeper each round.

When you land on the answer that stirs your heart with deep emotion-you've probably found your why (if not, you are closer then you were before).

Write it down. Put it on your mirror, in your gym bag, or on your phone background.

Challenge

- Share your *why* with a trusted brother, spouse, or mentor.
- Ask them to hold you accountable.

- Take one bold step this week aligned with your why:
    - Set a time for daily prayer.
    - Join the gym.
    - Set a new bedtime.
    - Say no to what doesn't serve your purpose.

Small steps with purpose beat big efforts without it.

Ask Holy Spirit daily: *"Does this support my purpose—or sabotage it?"*

Journal Prompts

- What has God put on my heart that I can no longer ignore?

- If I lived with my purpose in mind daily, what would I stop tolerating?

- If I lived with my purpose in mind daily, what would I start doing?

Closing Thought

Your *why* gives you energy when you want to quit. It helps you become the man God designed you to be: focused, faithful, and active in His Kingdom.

Jesus and the Power of Why

Hebrews 12:2 says Jesus endured the cross **for the joy set before Him**. That joy—our redemption—was His why. He didn't suffer because He loved pain. He suffered because He loved us. His purpose was redemption through the cross. His why was because He loved us.

When the journey gets painful—and it will—what is your "joy set before you" that will keep you in the fight?

Discover your Purpose, tap into your why, then live like it matters.

Chapter 6: Set the Right Goals

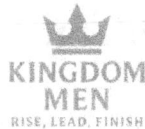

KINGDOM
MEN
RISE, LEAD, FINISH

Key Verses to Memorize:
"Write the vision and make it plain on tablets, that he may run who reads it." — *Habakkuk 2:2*

"Commit your works to the Lord, and your thoughts will be establish." — *Proverbs 16:3*

Now that you've discovered your *why*, it's time to make it crystal clear. Clarity is necessary to measure progress and we do this with goals. Goals are how we intentionally translate that clarity into action.

Establishing your *why* is a great step, but it will remain unfulfilled without an active strategy to see it realized in your life. Your *why* can serve as a filter through which you sift life's decisions. This filter helps ensure that your choices move you forward in the plans God has for you (**Ephesians 2:8–10**).

Men often experience decision fatigue when their *why* isn't firmly established, because life pulls them in so many different directions. Without settling the central question—*Which way am I going?*—they are left scattered and uncertain.

When your *why* is clear, it becomes the lens through which everything is filtered, making decision-making far more focused and efficient.

Vision without goals is just wishful thinking. Goals without God's vision for your life becomes a grind. But when vision and godly structure align, men move mountains.

Setting the right goals will help you build a structure that supports your calling—so you can run with endurance and finish strong.

Problem: Drift

Men drift when they have no direction. They coast, settle, and get soft.

We're not called to drift. We're called to move ahead on the path God has for us. We are to do so—with strength, focus, and precision.

To keep from drifting off course, sailors have relied on the stars. Those fixed points in the sky gave them direction, stability, and a way to measure their progress toward their destination. Without them, they could easily lose their way. In the same way, goals serve as markers for men. They keep us on course. They take our w*hy*—the reason we set out in the first place—and shape it into a straight, purposeful path.

Your w*hy* is your end goal, your big picture. It's the vision that gives meaning to the grind of each day. Yet this is where so many men falter. We get stuck in the weeds. We become overwhelmed by endless tasks, or we allow the small frustrations of life to cloud the bigger purpose. The details begin to dominate, and before long, we forget why we even started the journey.

That's why Scripture reminds us to look up: *"I lift up my eyes to the mountains—where does my help come from? My help comes from the Lord, the Maker of heaven and earth."* (**Psalm 121:1– 2**). When our eyes are fixed on God and His promises, we regain perspective. Isaiah paints a similar picture, calling us to lift our heads and see what God is doing (**Isaiah 49:18–23**). Only then can we properly align the small steps of our daily lives with the greater vision He has placed in our hearts.

Make it a habit to pause, look up, and remember where you're going. Let your w*hy* pull you forward. Then, organize your daily actions in a way that consistently moves you closer to that destination.

Never forget: God is for you. He is working all around you—even when you can't see it. But if your head stays buried in the obstacles, you will miss His perspective. You'll measure life only by its struggles instead of by His promises. And when that happens, you risk walking right past the abundant life He has planned for you.

The Problem with Vague Goals

Many men say things like, *"I just want to be healthier."* That's fine— but so does everyone. A desire without a plan is just wishful thinking. And when you live without clear goals, frustration is inevitable.

God wired men for the hunt. We need targets. We need something specific to pursue. Life isn't meant to be a casual hike; it's a mission, a pursuit, a chase after something that matters. Without that sense of pursuit, men drift. We lose direction. We settle for motion without progress.

Even Jesus lived with this kind of clarity. **Isaiah 50:7** says, God *"set His face like flint"* toward Jerusalem. He knew His destination. He understood His w*hy* and He moved with unwavering conviction and intentionality.

Here's the principle: if your goals don't serve your *purpose*, they don't just slow you down— they distract you. Instead of keeping you on course, they pull you off course. Instead of fueling your purpose, they drain your energy. That's why men who live without targets, or who chase the wrong ones, end up drifting through life instead of finishing their race with focus and strength.

Masculine Truth

A real man doesn't drift—he directs. He takes responsibility for his course. He creates structure, sets the pace, and embraces discipline. He doesn't just work hard; he works strategically.

Goals aren't about perfection. They're about progression. A man of God doesn't wait for life to magically improve—he builds. He sets goals that support his calling and strengthen his character. He pursues Kingdom goals, not hype. And those goals are forged in daily habits that eventually produce lasting fruit.

Training for the Fight

When I trained for bullfighting I couldn't just show up and hope things went well. My preparation was life-or-death. I had a plan:

- A workout schedule

- A nutrition plan

- Specific drills to build habits

- Film study/mental preperation

Every detail mattered, because my life—and the lives of others—depended on my preparation.

That's true for men today. What does your workout schedule look like? What is your nutrition plan? What specific daily habits are you intentionally building? What are you meditating on? Whatever it is, your meditation builds the pictures in your mind which you will live out. Take these things serious. Make a plan and execute it.

We don't need more *motivation*—we need *direction*. And not just vague direction, but one that's written down, prayed over, and pursued with intensity.

Motivation can help for a while. It's an outward push that moves us from comfort toward a goal. But once the external pressure fades, so does the drive. That's why so many men start strong but lose steam.

Inspiration, however, is different. Inspiration flows from within. As son's of God, Holy Spirit lives in us. He is our true source of power, urging us forward with strength that doesn't fade. If we find ourselves dependent only on motivation, it may be because we've ignored Holy Spirit's voice and settled for lesser substitutes. When that happens, it's time to repent and return to the One who truly fuels us from the inside out.

Motivation is external—it fades. Inspiration is internal—it flows from The Spirit.

Goals That Build, Not Burden

Once you know your w*hy*, it's time to build your h*ow*. Purpose without planning leads to frustration. Without direction, passion turns into burnout and potential remains untapped. And truthfully, a man without a plan eventually becomes a burden to those around him. Proverbs warns, "Whoever falsely boasts of giving is like clouds and wind without rain" (**Proverbs 25:14**). In other words, empty promises and unfulfilled potential create disappointment instead of blessing.

Spiritual Insight: God Is a Planner

Planning is not unspiritual—it's biblical. God is a planner. He created the world with order and structure. He designed the body with systems.

He gave Noah blueprints for the ark. He gave David battle strategies. Even Jesus followed a divine timetable, moving with intentionality toward His mission.

When God told Noah to build the ark, He didn't simply say, "Build a boat." He gave precise dimensions (**Genesis 6:14–16**). That's because God is specific. And He calls His men to be the same.

Setting goals is not merely a productivity exercise—it's an act of worship. It's stewardship. It's how we align ourselves with God's wisdom and partner with Holy Spirit to build something that lasts.

The SMART Way to Set Goals

Stop saying "someday." *Someday* isn't on the calendar. A Kingdom man doesn't wait for a better season—he starts now. He sets goals, invites Holy Spirit to lead him, and takes responsibility for his direction.

Sometimes, the most spiritual thing you can do is the most practical. Godly men don't separate prayer from planning. They seek God's presence and then build according to His wisdom.

One of the simplest, time-tested frameworks for goal-setting is called **SMART goals**. When filtered through Kingdom stewardship, it becomes a powerful tool:

- **Specific** – Define exactly what you are building.

- **Measurable** – If you can't track it, you can't improve it.

- **Attainable** – It should stretch you, but not break you.

- **Realistic** – Ask: is this doable in this season?

- **Time-sensitive** – Deadlines create discipline.

Example:" I will work out three times per week at 7 a.m. for the next 30 days to build strength and energy for my calling."

Notice: the goal is clear, practical, and tied to a w*hy*. Your goals should always serve your purpose—not replace it.

Core Ideas

- A vague vision produces scattered results.

- Without structure, passion turns into pressure.

- The best goals grow you and glorify God.

- Planning is spiritual—it's a form of worship.

Questions to Ask Yourself

- Where am I vague or aimless in my life?

- What area needs structure to support my vision?

- Are my goals aligned with my calling—or are they just reactive?

- If I stay on this trajectory, where will I end up?

- Do my goals excite and challenge me—or do they leave me anxious and overwhelmed?

- What obstacles tend to derail me—and what's my plan when they show up?

- What single goal, if pursued for 90 days, would change my life?

Action: Draft Your First SMART Goal

Pick one key area of your life:

- Spiritual

- Physical

- Financial

- Relational

- Emotional

Now write your first SMART goal.

Example:" I will wake up at 6 a.m. to spend 30 minutes in prayer and Scripture five days a week for the next 30 days."

Then go deeper:

- What could derail me?

- What habit will I need to build?

- What reward will I set?

Write it. Schedule it. Tell someone.

Challenge

Put your goal somewhere visible:

- Sticky note on the mirror

- Phone lock screen

- Calendar alert

Each morning, read it. Declare it. Act on it.

Men of God don't drift to greatness—they intentionally direct their lives. They *write the vision, make it plain, and run with purpose* (**Habakkuk 2:2**). Set your goals. Then go to war.

The best goals are not only clear and measurable—they're shared. Tell your wife. Tell your brother. Tell your small group. Accountability isn't weakness—it's wisdom. It makes you a Kingdom man who refuses to walk alone. Share your goal, and ask for prayer and follow-up.

Journal Prompts

- If I don't set goals in this season, where will I drift—and what will it cost?

- What have I failed to build because I never set clear goals?

- Where do I need more structure?

- What's one small goal that would create big change over time?

Closing Thought

Goals without God lead to pride. God without goals leads to passivity. But a man who walks with God *and* sets Spirit-led goals? That man moves mountains.

You are not here to live lukewarm. You are here to live laser-focused on your calling. Let your goals reflect the weight of your *Purpose*. **Set the goals. Then go to war.**

Chapter 7: Unity of Spirit, Soul, and Body

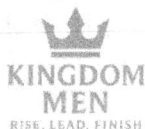

KINGDOM
MEN
RISE, LEAD, FINISH

Key Verses to Memorize:

"May your whole spirit, soul and body be preserved blameless at the
coming of our Lord Jesus Christ." — **1 Thessalonians 5:23**

"Be transformed by the renewing of your mind." — **Romans 12:2**

God's Design for Wholeness

God designed you as a whole man—spirit, soul, and body. When those
three parts are aligned under the lordship of Christ, you become
powerful, stable, and dangerous to darkness.

A divided man is a vulnerable man. But a united man is an unstoppable force.

Wholeness is not about perfection—it's about unity. God doesn't want just part of you. He wants all of you—spirit, soul, and body—aligned, ordered, and ready for mission.

Unfortunately, we have lost much of this unity. We tend to separate the spiritual from the physical, ranking them in an unsupported hierarchy where the "spiritual" is important, but the physical is optional—or even irrelevant. That mindset robs us of power. As long as we treat the physical world as though it isn't spiritual, we will never fully experience the Kingdom in our life as God intended on this side of eternity.

Remember **Genesis 2:7** God formed man's physical body in His image (**Genesis 1:26–27**). Jesus Himself took on a physical body as part of redemption (**Philippians 2:7**). He was beaten and crucified to bring healing to your body (**Isaiah 53:5**). God values your body—He created it, Jesus redeemed it, and the Spirit dwells in it. The question is: do you value it the same way?

Unity Defined

You can eat clean, work out, and still feel stuck. Why? Because health doesn't start in your biceps—it starts in your being.

When a man is divided within himself—saying one thing, doing another and believing something else—he loses his authority. Disunity leads to dysfunction. Unity leads to strength.

God created you as a triune (3 part) being:

- **Spirit** – the eternal breath of life God breathed into mankind (**Genesis 2:7**) that must be born again to see the kingdom of God- (**John 3:3**).
  Spirit exists in the Spirit Realm and is influenced by and influences the natural realm.

- **Soul** – your mind, will, and emotions.
  Conduit between the spirit realm and physical realm.

- **Body** – your physical vessel, the temple of the Holy Spirit.
  Exists in the spirt realm.

Too many men live out of only one part. Some are soul-driven, reacting to every emotion. Others are body-driven, ruled by cravings, comfort, or vanity. Few are truly spirit-led—living with alignment and power.

When your spirit leads, your soul submits, and your body follows. That is wholeness.

Masculine Truth

Strength comes from unity. Disorder is not manly—it's immature. Fragmentation opens the door to distraction, addiction, and deception.

A man aligned—spirit strong, soul healed, and body disciplined—is a man of resilience, wisdom, and trustworthiness. You weren't made to live scattered. You were built to live from a united heart: spirit-led, emotionally grounded, and physically prepared.

Biblical Anchor: Jesus in the Wilderness

Before launching His public ministry, Jesus spent 40 days in the wilderness—fasting, praying, resisting temptation. That wasn't just spiritual preparation—it was physical, emotional, and mental discipline.

And the result? Scripture says He returned *"in the power of the Spirit"* (**Luke 4:14**). Unity within produced power for the mission of establishing His Kingdom.

The Problem with Fragmented Living

Here's what fragmentation sounds like with an unrenewed mind:

- *"I want health but don't know if God wants me healed"* —(soul).

- *"I want to keep binge eating"* —(body).

- *"I don't believe I'm worth healing"*—(spirit).

That's a man at war with himself. He says one thing, does another, and believes something entirely different.

We need to bring our body and soul into submission under the leading of Holy Spirit. Fragmentation causes burnout. Unity produces breakthrough.

A Kingdom Man in Alignment

Now flip the script:

- His spirit declares: *"God wants me whole."*

- His soul agrees: *"I choose thoughts that align with truth."* (**2 Corinthians 10:5**)

- His body acts: *"I will honor God with my choices. I will present my body as a living sacrifice, holy and acceptable to God."* (**Romans 12:1**)

That's the man who becomes unstoppable—not just in physical health, but in leadership, marriage, and calling.

Core Ideas

- Your spirit, soul, and body are individual parts, intertwined to make a whole.

- Ignoring one weakens the others.

- Your spirit should lead your soul, and your soul should lead your body in submission to Christ.

- Disunity creates dysfunction. Unity produces power.

The Power of a Renewed Mind

Romans 12:2 commands us to be transformed by the renewing of our mind. That's your soul— the seat of thought, decision, and emotion.

Your soul is where truth is either accepted or rejected. It's where the battle is won or lost. You may believe in healing, but if your thoughts and emotions aren't renewed, you will default to old patterns of thinking and doing.

- If your thoughts remain unrenewed, you will sabotage progress. For example, *continuing to walk in unforgiveness, bitterness and anger. Verbally agreeing with the lies of the enemy and thus opening doors into your life for the enemy to enter, or habitually eating junk food.*

- If your emotions lead, your habits will follow dysfunction.

- But if your soul submits to the Spirit, you'll walk in lasting change.

Action: Soul Inventory

Consider your answers honestly:

- What thoughts dominate my day-to-day life? i.e. *pornography, self-doubt, anxiety, worry,* fear etc.

- Which part of me does most of the leading—spirit, soul, or body?

- Where am I living divided?

- What physical habits are opposing my spiritual convictions?

- What would wholeness look like for me in this season?

- What emotions typically drive my actions?

- Do my choices reflect a man led by the Spirit—or by my feelings?

Then invite Holy Spirit to speak truth into each area. Write it down. Declare it out loud.

Key Verse to Memorize:
"Bless the Lord, O my soul, and all that is within me, bless His holy name." — **Psalm 103:1**

David spoke to his soul and brought it into alignment with truth. You must do the same.

Challenge: A Full Audit

Pick one day this week for a full audit of your life:

- **Spirit** – How aware am I of God's presence throughout the day?

- **Soul** – How are my thoughts and emotions aligning with truth?

- **Body** – How am I honoring God with what I eat, how I move, and how I rest?

Ask yourself: *"Where am I thriving? Where am I drifting?"*
Then schedule one intentional step to restore unity.

Journal Prompts

- Where have I lived fragmented—and what will I do to become whole again?

- What does wholeness look like in this season?

- What daily practices bring unity—or create disunity—in my life?

Closing Thought

You are not just a man in a body. You are a spirit-filled, soul-restored, physically equipped son in the Kingdom of God.

God doesn't want part of you—He wants all of you. Aligned. Ordered. Ready.

When your whole self—spirit, soul, and body—comes under the lordship of Christ, you don't just survive. You take dominion.

Wholeness is possible, and it doesn't happen by accident. Unity is powerful.

Get aligned. Get activated. Get after it. Because a united man is an unstoppable force.

Chapter 8: Balance Without Compromise

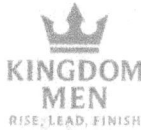

KINGDOM
MEN
RISE, LEAD, FINISH

Key Verses to Memorize:

"Dishonest scales are an abomination to the Lord, but a just weight is His delight." — **Proverbs 11:1**

"Let your eyes look straight ahead; fix your gaze directly before you. Give careful thought to the paths for your feet and be steadfast in all your ways." — **Proverbs 4:25–26** (NIV)

"Be still, and know that I am God." — **Psalm 46:10**

God's Design for Balance

Balance isn't soft—it's strategic. Too many men hear the word "balance" and think it means slowing down, doing less, or playing it safe. But Kingdom balance isn't about comfort. It's about clarity, order, and faithfulness.

Balance is knowing what matters most and giving it the right weight. It's not about avoiding responsibility, but about aligning your life with God's priorities.

If the enemy can't destroy you, he'll distract you. If he can't stop you, he'll burn you out. But when a man is balanced under God's order, he isn't stretched thin—he's strengthened. He isn't scattered—he's sharp.

Biblical balance is not passive. It's powerful.

The Suzuki in Dubois

I was driving about 35 mph on my way out of Dubois, a sleepy little town in eastern Idaho, when my little Suzuki Swift started bouncing around like a busted carnival ride. I slowed down and it went away. When I sped up, it started jack rabbiting around again which made me think I had hit washboards in the road, so I stopped to give it the once over. But when I stopped to check it out, I realized a weight on the rear wheel had shifted just enough to throw an egg shaped wobble in my tire. It was out of balance.

It wasn't the road. It was my balance.

Life works the same way. Without balance, things quickly get chaotic, wobble, shake, and eventually break down.

The Problem: Why Most Men Fail Here

Men don't usually fall because of weakness—they fall because of imbalance.

- Too much work, not enough rest.

- All discipline, no joy.

- 100% performance, 0% presence.

- Pouring out, but never receiving.

- Serving others, without wisdom.

Most men live out of balance. They ignore the warning signs and keep driving until the damage is done. The tragedy isn't just imbalance itself—it's refusing to pull over and make the adjustment.

There's a principle called the Pareto Principle, or the 80/20 rule. An economist discovered that roughly 80% of results come from just 20% of the causes. This principle helps us prioritize our efforts by focusing on the small portion that produces the greatest impact.

We all have the same 24 hours in a day, so we must use them wisely. We can spend our time trying to improve our weaknesses, or we can invest that same time in sharpening our strengths. Each of us has unique gifts and callings we naturally excel in, as well as areas where we struggle. When I focus on my strengths, the time I invest produces multiplied results. But when I focus on my weaknesses, the return is minimal. The difference isn't in the hours spent—it's in the impact those hours create. The greatest impact comes from focusing our efforts on what matters most.

Masculine Truth

Balance isn't about doing less—it's about doing what matters most, consistently.

The most dangerous men aren't the busiest or most talented. They're the most disciplined. The most ordered.

A Kingdom man doesn't hustle out of fear, trying to prove himself, or slack-off out of laziness and passivity. He walks in rhythm with God. The world says, *"Do it all."* God says, *"Do what* matters."

You can't lead with conviction if your energy is being burned up by what doesn't matter. Balance leads to overflow. Imbalance leads to exhaustion.

Biblical Anchor: The Pace of Jesus

Look at the life of Jesus. He never rushed. Never panicked. Never burned out. He was the most powerful man to ever walk the earth, and He lived with intentional rhythm.

- He withdrew often to pray—**Luke 5:16**.

- He said no to distractions.—**Luke 10:38-42**, **Matthew 8:21-22**.

- He responded to urgency with peace, not pressure—**Mark 4:39**.

- In storms, He slept—**Mark 4:38**.

- In crisis, He **waited** for the Father's timing—**John 11:1-44**.

Consider the storm on the Sea of Galilee: the disciples panicked, but Jesus spoke peace. Or the death of Lazarus: Martha was frantic, but Jesus moved in God's timing, not human urgency. He wasn't reactive. He was intentionally *responsive*.

Jesus was intense—He overturned tables and rebuked demons—but He also retreated often to be with the Father (**Luke 5:16**). He lived in divine rhythm, never letting the urgent override the important.

That's balance. That's Kingdom leadership.

If the Son of God needed rest, rhythm, and retreat—so do you. How are you doing with that?

The word *"wait"* in **Isaiah 40:31** doesn't imply passivity. It means *"to bind together, to gather, to* tarry patiently, to wait for, or to wait on." It's active, not idle.

When Scripture tells us to *wait on the Lord,* picture a waiter at a restaurant. A good waiter doesn't change your order because he thinks you'd like something else better. He doesn't pass your order off to another server because he doesn't agree with your request. He simply receives your instructions and faithfully carries them out.

In the same way, when we wait on the Father's timing, we are actively obeying what He's already commanded us to do. He's given you an assignment—your job is to serve, to trust, and to follow through.

But many men struggle here. We tend to take matters into our own hands when God's timeline doesn't match ours. We act prematurely, driven by impatience rather than faith. Just like Abraham, who chose to bring about God's promise through Hagar instead of waiting for Sarah, we try to manufacture the right outcome in the wrong way.

And while our way might look productive, it's rarely aligned with His purpose.

Coach's Corner: Order Creates Overflow

Balance doesn't mean every area of life gets equal time. It means every area gets its rightful place.

When Jesus was asked about the greatest commandment, He answered, *"You shall love the Lord* your God with all your heart, soul, and mind... and love your neighbor as yourself"* (**Matthew 22:37–39**). Notice: the second command flows out of the first. Love for God becomes love expressed to others.

Most men see life as a vertical priority list:

1. God

2. Spouse

3. Children

4. Brotherhood (Church/Community)

5. Work/Calling

But it's more accurate to see it as a foundation. God is the source of love that flows into every other relationship and responsibility. Balance means allowing His love to guide how you steward your wife, children, work, and all He has entrusted to you.

When the foundation is honored, your life gains harmony. But when it's ignored, you end up replacing God with yourself—and eventually, you'll be crushed under the weight of your own efforts.

Balance means saying *no* with wisdom, *yes* with conviction, and leading from overflow—not depletion.

The Dangers of Extremes

Balance isn't 50/50. It's about right weight in the right place.

You're not meant to spend equal time in the gym and in the Word. But you are meant to steward both according to your season and assignment.

Even good things—when taken to excess—can throw you off balance. Too much of one thing can keep you from the one thing God is actually asking of you.

Balance keeps the wheels rolling smoothly, with power and purpose.

Practical Signs You're Out of Balance

- You're constantly tired or short-tempered.

- You struggle to hear clearly from God.

- You feel guilty whenever you rest.

- Your calendar dictates your life.

- You haven't spent un-rushed time with family.

- Your health is declining despite your effort.

Core Ideas

- God honors order.

- Balance isn't static—it's a moving rhythm, not a rigid formula.

- When you lead from balance, you lead with clarity and peace.

- What you prioritize reveals what you truly value.

- You don't have to do everything—just what matters.

- Don't confuse motion with mission.

- Stillness is strength—when it's submitted to God.

- Sons don't hustle for approval. They receive from the Father and move with purpose.

Questions

- Where am I out of balance—and how is it effecting those I lead?

- What distractions are distorting my focus and consuming time that should be invested in my calling?

- Am I reacting to life—or intentionally ordering it?

- Have I confused burnout with serving?

Action: Create a Balance Audit

Draw a simple pie chart. Label five areas:

- Spiritual

- Physical

- Mental/Emotional

- Relational

- Financial

Now evaluate the past seven days. Where did your time and energy go? Are your investments aligned with your values? Where is there excess—or neglect?

Look at your calendar, in light of your habits and energy.

- What needs to be scheduled with priority?

Then ask Holy Spirit:

- "Where do You want me to shift my weight?"

- "What do I need to remove to make room for what matters?"

Write it down. Then obey.

If you're unsure what He's saying, start here until clarity comes:

- Begin your days with prayer

- Prioritize your relationships

- Work with focus

- Rest without guilt

This is what Kingdom balance looks like. Balance isn't about "having it all"—it's about stewarding well what you've been given. God isn't impressed with your pace. He desires your presence.

Challenge: Fight for Rhythmic Living

God built the world in rhythms:

- Day and night

- Seedtime and harvest

- Work and Sabbath

Kingdom men learn to live by divine rhythm, not worldly hustle.

This week, choose one area where you've overextended yourself. Ask: *Why?* What's driving you to choose works over grace? Invite Jesus into that space to heal the root issue. Then, reallocate that time toward simple obedience.

- Sabbath rest

- Worship

- Quality time with your wife/kids

- Un-rushed prayer

- Physical movement

- Study in the Word

Men will often look at rest as unproductive. Remember what God Says in **Psalm 46:10**, "Be still and know that I am God". He is not asking. This is a command. Don't call it unproductive. Call it obedience.

Journal Prompts

- Where am I letting life dictate my priorities instead of God?

- What would it look like to live from peace and order, not pressure and chaos?

- What is the real cost of imbalance in my life?

- How would my leadership change if I led from balance instead of burnout?

- What small shift would create the biggest clarity and capacity?

Closing Thought

You are not a machine. You are not a slave to hustle. You are a son.

Balance isn't weakness. It is not compromise. Balance is strength under order. It's living in rhythm with God.

Live ordered. Live aligned. Live dangerous to the darkness.

Chapter 9: Train Like a Fighter

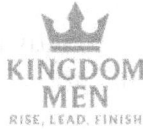

Key Verses to Memorize:

"Discipline yourself for the purpose of godliness. For physical training is of some value, but godliness has value for all things..." —
1 Timothy 4:7–8 (NIV)

"Do you not know that those who run in a race all run, but one receives the prize? Run in such away that you may obtain it."
— 1 Corinthians 9:24

"I discipline my body and bring it under subjection, lest, when I have preached to others, I myself should become disqualified."
— 1 Corinthians 9:27

God's Design: Men were Made for War

A Kingdom man doesn't train for comfort—he trains for combat. Training isn't about six-pack abs or personal records in the gym. It's about building strength for your assignment.

Men of God are called to treat their lives like a mission. That means training intentionally— cultivating habits that build endurance, resilience, and readiness in every area: spiritual, physical, emotional, financial, and relational.

Men need to have the discipline to cultivate the habits and mindset that produce strength, endurance, and grit.

Discipline isn't comfortable and it isn't punishment. It's preparation. And preparation is the foundation for success (Dr. Edwin Louis Cole).

When God created Adam, He didn't place him in a garden filled with ease—He placed him in a raw, untamed wilderness. Then He gave him a mission: *take dominion and subdue it.*

From the beginning, man was designed to come alive in challenge. Work wasn't a curse—it was part of his calling. Adam's job was to bring order to the chaos, to rule over God's creation and draw out its potential. As he did, the wild became fruitful. The untamed became useful. Provision followed purpose.

But here's the pattern: as men bring creation under control, we tend to make life more comfortable—roads, cities, homes, climate control. The list goes on and on. Though things that bring comfort are not inherently wrong, they come with a cost.

Over time, comfort makes men soft.

Instead of ruling over creation, we become ruled by comfort. The very things we built to serve us begin to control us. We trade dominion for convenience and authority for ease. Too often, men stop subduing—and start settling.

Bullfighting and Battle Readiness

During my bullfighting career, there was no room for laziness. If I was out of shape, someone could get hurt—or worse. My training wasn't optional. I worked my legs, lungs, reflexes, and mind. I stayed clear-headed and sharp, because lives depended on it.

The same is true outside the arena. The discipline that saves lives in the arena is the same discipline that saves marriages, fights for those who cannot protect themselves, guards purity, and protects your calling.

The question is: are you training for your calling—or coasting through peacetime? If you fail to subdue and take dominion, you will get soft and become an easy target for the enemy.

The Problem: Weakness and Passivity

Lazy men don't change the world. Weak men don't protect families. Passive men don't stand against darkness.

Here's the truth: the enemy doesn't fear your intentions—he fears your preparation. Too many men rely on motivation, but motivation fades. Masculinity doesn't wait for the mood to strike— men train whether they feel like it or not. Men train with intention.

Without daily discipline, your body becomes a liability, your soul becomes unstable, and your spirit becomes dull. And when that happens, you can't lead your family, fight for the Kingdom, or walk in the fullness of your calling. If you want to be sharp in your mind, strong in your body, and steady in your soul—you must train. Not once. Not occasionally. Daily. Intentionally.

Masculine Truth

Masculinity calls a man to train even when no one is watching. Masculine men live ready.

- A man doesn't train for self—he trains for the mission-to guide, guard and govern others.

- Your discipline proves how seriously you take your mission.

- Weak men wait for motivation. Kingdom men train with intention.

- Training isn't occasional—it's daily. It's deliberate. It's decisive.

God Gives Us His Strength

Scripture consistently highlights strength:

- David fought lions, bears, and giants.

- Samson defeated armies with a jawbone.

- Jesus endured the cross after being brutally beaten.

- Paul survived shipwrecks and stonings, yet he pressed forward.

Strength is not optional for Kingdom men. You were created to be a pillar of strength in your family, church, and community. But strength without surrender is dangerous. Plenty of strong men have destroyed marriages, wounded children, and lost control of themselves (**Proverbs 7:26**). Godly strength is different— it's strength under submission.

"The meek shall inherit the earth" (**Matthew 5:5**). Meekness means strength under control. A godly man trains his body to serve his purpose—not replace it. Keep this in order.

Kingdom Fitness: A Reframe

Physical fitness is not vanity—it's spiritual warfare.
Why? Because when you're tired, sick, or weak, it becomes harder to:

- Be patient with your kids

- Focus in prayer

- Show up at work

- Serve with joy

- Discern God's voice

Training your body is an act of stewardship. It ensures your body doesn't become a limitation to your calling.

Coach's Corner: Three Training Arenas

Every man needs to train in three arenas:

- **Spirit** – Word, prayer, worship, fasting

- **Soul** – Mindset, focus, emotional awareness, humility, willpower

- **Body** – Nutrition/hydration, movement, strength, sleep, recovery

Neglect one, and the other two will suffer. You don't need a fancy gym or endless time. You need a plan—and a reason. Train for the man you're becoming, not the man you used to be.

Practical Framework: Five Pillars of Masculine Training

1. Function First – Train with movements that matter: squats, carries, lunges, push-ups, sprints. Build strength that lasts.

2. Consistency Over Intensity – Twenty minutes a day beats two hours once a week. Master your schedule.

3. Fuel Like a Fighter – Eat for energy, not escape. Prioritize whole foods and hydration. Eliminate processed junk.

4. Rest and Rebuild – You grow in recovery. Sleep is spiritual. Prioritize it.

5. Discipline the Mind – Motivation dies. Disciplined inspiration endures. Don't wait to feel like it.

Core Ideas

- Physical Training is stewardship, not vanity.

- Your body is a tool, not your master.

- You don't need to be shredded—you need to be ready.

- The enemy preys on unprepared men.

- Train for the man you're becoming—not the man you've been.

Questions

- How am I training my body to support my calling?

- Can my body keep up with my calling?

- Where am I undisciplined—and what is it costing me?

- What daily practices would sharpen my edge?

- Am I preparing for war—or coasting through peacetime?

- Am I training to glorify God—or impress people?

- Do I glorify God in how I eat, train, and recover?

- What would my family or team say about my discipline?

Action: Set a Masculine Rhythm

Design your weekly rhythm to train like a fighter. Include:

- **Physical Movement**: 3–5x/week

- **Spiritual Discipline: Word and prayer daily**

- **Mental Sharpening: Journaling, reading, limiting distractions**

Make it non-negotiable. Block it on your calendar. Journal what shifts. Treat it like your life depends on it—because it does.

Challenge: The Masculine Week

This week, commit to five straight days of:

- **Move**: At least 20 minutes of training (walk, lift, stretch, sprint).

- **Fuel**: Eat only what serves your strength and mission.

- **Speak**: Declare daily strength over yourself—be excellent in your speech all day everyday.

Example Declarations:

- "My body is the temple of the living God; I honor God with it.

- "I was made strong for a purpose.

- " I train today for battles I haven't even seen yet."

Write your own. Speak it until you believe it.

Journal Prompts

- If I trained for my calling like a fighter trains for battle, how would my life look different?

- Where have I lacked discipline—and what has it cost me?

- What would change if I trained daily like my life and mission depended on it?

- What story do I want my strength to tell?

Closing Thought

Weak men wait for motivation. Masculine men are not concerned with motivation, they train in the dark so they can lead in the light.

You weren't made to sit the bench. You were made to advance the Kingdom.

Train like your life depends on it—because it does.

Chapter 10: Fast and Fight

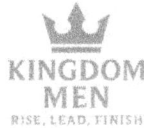

KINGDOM
MEN
RISE, LEAD, FINISH

Key Verses to Memorize:

"When you fast, do not be like the hypocrites… But you, when you fast, anoint your head and wash your face, so that you do not appear to men to be fasting…" — **Matthew 6:16–18**

"Is this not the fast that I have chosen: to loose the bonds of wickedness, to undo heavy burdens, to let the oppressed go free, and that you break every yoke?" — **Isaiah 58:6**

"Man shall not live by bread alone, but by every word that proceeds from the mouth of God." — **Matthew 4:4**

"I am the bread of life."—**John 6:35**

God's Design: Fasting as a Weapon

Spiritual warfare requires strategy. Fasting is a battle tactic, not a diet. It's not about deprivation —it's about dominion.

Kingdom men deny the flesh to hear the Father. They understand that fasting sharpens clarity, multiplies power, and restores authority. Fasting is a forgotten weapon, often ignored or misunderstood. We talk about prayer. We teach on worship. But fasting? Most men avoid it— either because they don't understand it or they lack the discipline to do it.

Yet, notice Jesus 'words: *"When you fast"* (**Matthew 6:16**). Not *if*. **When**. For Kingdom men, fasting is not optional—it's expected.

Fasting isn't about showmanship. It's not about appearing spiritual. It's about sharpening your edge. It's about starving the flesh so your spirit can see and hear. Fasting quiets the noise, awakens clarity, and restores strength for battle.

You don't fight spiritual battles with fleshly weapons. You fight with a life of worship which includes; prayer, truth, and fasting. Fasting is the intentional surrender of the physical to strengthen the spiritual. It's how Kingdom men fight unseen battles.

My Introduction to Fasting

When I first began fasting, it was out of obedience and for health reasons. But what surprised me most was how it sharpened my spirit.

I began to notice how often I reached for food out of habit, boredom, or stress. Fasting created space—and that space led to greater dependency on God. My prayers became sharper. My mind clearer. My spirit stronger.

Jesus modeled fasting before His mission. I discovered it wasn't about deprivation—it was about alignment. Fasting didn't just help me physically, it realigned me with God in a way nothing else had.

Obedience—not outcome—brings the blessing.

The Problem: Why Men Avoid Fasting

Fasting and Obedience

Interestingly, in **Luke 18** the Pharisee mentions fasting twice a week in the same breath as tithing. Most of us recognize the blessing of obedience in giving—but skip right over the discipline of fasting. Could it be that fasting was assumed to be part of a believer's lifestyle? Perhaps that's why Jesus said *"when you fast"*—because His audience already understood its place in a life of obedience.

Obedience matters more than outcome. We may not always know the "why" behind God's instructions, but our responsibility is to obey. Fasting is a clear example. The blessing isn't in the results we expect—it's in the obedience itself.

Beyond Religious Showmanship

Too often, fasting is misunderstood. Some treat it as a religious performance, assuming that skipping meals or enduring hunger will somehow make them more spiritual. But this misses the point.

Fasting is not about self-deprivation. It's about making space. It's not just about giving something up—it's about entering rest and alignment with God.

I've always wrestled with the idea that fasting is simply about replacing mealtimes with prayer or Bible reading. While those are good practices, fasting is more than a rigid spiritual exchange.

Done with the wrong heart, it can become as empty as the rituals of people who crucify themselves during Holy Week in an effort to prove devotion. That's not God's design.

Holy Spirit constantly reminds us with words like *grace, freedom, acceptance, righteousness, and peace.* Fasting is not about earning God's love. It's about living in the love and freedom He has already given.

Grace, Not Works

Though most Christians would affirm that salvation is by grace through faith, many still live as though grace is only partially effective—and we must add "spiritual gymnastics" to earn God's favor. Fasting, when misunderstood, can fall into this trap.

But what if fasting is less about trying to earn spiritual points, and more about cultivating a disciplined lifestyle? What if it's as practical as it is spiritual—removing physical burdens so that our minds are clearer, our hearts are purified, and our lives are better aligned with God's will?

Remember: *"Keep your heart with all diligence, for out of it spring the issues of life."* (**Proverbs 4:23**) Fasting creates space for clarity, which purifies the heart, which in turn aligns our lives more closely with His will.

God's Design for the Body

Science actually affirms what Scripture teaches. Our bodies were designed to thrive when cared for with wisdom and discipline.

For example, the body functions best in what's called the **parasympathetic state**—a state of rest, digestion, and rebuilding. In this state, nutrients are properly absorbed, food is digested well, and the body recovers. But constant eating, stress, or overindulgence keeps us in a **sympathetic state**—the familiar "fight or flight" mode.

God even designed a process called the **Migrating Motor Complex (MMC)**, which sends wave- like motions through the small intestine every 15 minutes to clear out bacteria and keep the body clean. The catch? It only works when we're in a fasted state. Eating constantly turns this cleaning cycle off. If you snack all day, you never allow your body to "clean house" and as such, you become burdened down with toxins and inflammation.

So here's the question: how long has it been since you let your body clean house?

Neglecting the Body and Tempting God

Here's a hard truth: many of us treat our bodies recklessly, then ask God to miraculously fix the damage. How many times have you grabbed a donut in the church foyer without thinking of the impact on your health? How often do you pray *"by His stripes I am healed"* while continuing to abuse your body with junk food, caffeine overloads, and stress?

Scripture warns us: *"It has been said, you shall not tempt the Lord your God"* (**Luke 4:12**). Yet we do it when we neglect stewardship of our bodies and then expect God to bail us out when we refuse to walk a disciplined lifestyle.

Patterns and Principles

Throughout Scripture, God operates by patterns and principles. Take finances as an example. Financial health isn't a mystery—it comes by practicing stewardship, living within your means, learning your craft, and trusting God with tithes and offerings. Our responsibility pairs with His provision to produce blessing.

The same is true with health. Many believers expect God to handle all aspects of healing while they neglecting diet, exercise, rest, and emotional health. As Dr. David Perlmutter put it: *"We live in a society that tends to support the notion that we can live our lives however we choose and then, when we suddenly develop a health issue, there will be some powerful medical approach that will put us back on our feet."*

Sadly, the same mindset exists in the church. Many eat poorly, neglect movement, carry unforgiveness and bitterness, and then wonder why they're sick or burned out. When healing doesn't come instantly, they blame God.

Fasting realigns this imbalance. It reminds us that health is not magic—it's stewardship. God's power is made available through our obedience.

Most men avoid fasting because:

• It feels meaningless.

• It doesn't produce immediate results.

• It disrupts comfort.

• It challenges control.

But that's the point. You can't walk in Kingdom authority while being a slave to cravings. If food—or comfort—rules you, you're not free. And if you're not free, you can't lead others into freedom.

Immature men treat fasting like a religious ritual or a performance. It is dismissed as outdated and unnecessary. They treat their body carelessly, praying for healing while fueling themselves with junk food, stress, and neglect.

Fasting exposes all of that. It reveals who's really in charge—your flesh or your spirit.

Masculine Truth

Fasting builds control. It cultivates authority. Every time you fast, you tell your flesh: *"You don't run this house. Holy Spirit does."*

- Fasting builds self-control.

- Fasting starves pride.

- Fasting silences the flesh.

- Fasting prepares you for assignments in a way comfort never could.

We must be led by the Spirit and the flesh must follow. You can't walk in Kingdom authority while being a slave to your cravings. We don't fast to earn God's love. We don't fast to prove our spirituality. We fast out of obedience. And obedience brings blessing.

Biblical Anchor: Jesus in the Wilderness

Before launching His public ministry, Jesus fasted for 40 days. Why? Because fasting prepares you for battle.

- Before He healed the sick, He fasted.

- Before He cast out demons, He fasted.

- Before He preached to the crowds, He fasted.

Fasting preceded power.

"Then Jesus was led up by the Spirit into the wilderness to be tempted by the devil. And after fasting forty days and forty nights, He was hungry" (**Matthew 4:1–2**).

Jesus entered the wilderness in obedience and left in the power of the Spirit.

If the Son of God needed fasting to prepare for His mission—so do you.

The Solution: Fasting for Breakthrough

Isaiah 58 declares that true fasting *"looses the bonds of wickedness… breaks every yoke."* Fasting is not just personal—it's corporate. Your fasting can bring breakthrough for your wife, your children, and your church.

Fasting accomplishes what willpower never could. Fasting:

*   Breaks addictions

*   Sharpens discernment

*   Restores hunger for God

*   Kills passivity

*   Unlocks spiritual authority

*   Makes space for clarity

Fasting starves the flesh, training you to have self-control which brings your body under subjection to the Spirit. It increases sensitivity to Holy Spirit. And it makes space for clarity.

Some mountains simply won't move without fasting. When the disciples couldn't cast out a demon, Jesus said plainly: "This kind can come out by nothing but prayer and fasting" (**Mark 9:29**). Fasting is necessary, NOT optional.

Types of Fasts

Choose a fast with purpose:

- **Sun-Up to Sun-Down Fast** – Eat only after sunset. A great place to start.

- **24-Hour Fast** – Skip all meals. Use the time for prayer and worship.

- **3 Day fast from food, only drink Water**– For breakthrough, not for show.

Fasting without focus is just a diet. Tie your fast to prayer, worship, and obedience.

Coach's Corner: Practical Wisdom

- Fasting doesn't earn you more of God—it gives God more of you.

- Start small. Be intentional. Make it meaningful.

- Replace meals with Scripture, prayer, or stillness.

- Don't fast just to "get something." Fast to become the kind of man God can trust with more.

- Fast out of submission and obedience to God's word.
- Fasting isn't the absence of eating—it is taking dominion of the flesh in obedience.

- Fasting without focus is just a diet. The blessing is not in the result—it's in your obedience.

Core Ideas

- Fasting is spiritual warfare. With it we win unseen battles.

- The Spirit must lead; the flesh must follow.

- Fasting builds spiritual clarity, humility, healing, and authority.

- We don't fast to earn God's love—we fast because we are already loved.

- Real men deny the flesh to hear the Father.

- Fasting is obedience, not legalism.

Questions

- What comforts have become crutches in my life?

- What breakthrough am I praying for—but not preparing for?

- Where is my flesh too loud?

- Am I willing to sacrifice comfort to gain clarity?

- What area of life needs less clutter and more God?

- What's blurring my focus—and am I willing to fast to fix it?

Action: Choose a Fast

*all information I recommend on fasting is just that, a recommendation. You must make your own decision on how you fast and if you fast.

If this is your first time fasting, pick one of these fasts this week:

- Intermittent (skip breakfast)

- Sun-Up to Sun-Down fast

- 24-Hour fast

During your fast:

- Write down the specific breakthrough you are fasting for.

- Replace mealtime with prayer or worship.

- Journal what God is refining in you.

Challenge: 3-Day Fast

Get your strategy together so you can successfully do a three days fast:

1. Write down the breakthrough you're believing for.

2. Every time hunger hits, pray with authority.

3. Spend 15 minutes daily-put on worship music to engage with God.

4. Expect God to speak. Expect clarity. Expect resistance— and expect to push through.

Don't just skip meals. Go to war.

Journal Prompts

- Where is my flesh too loud? Most will jump to, "I'm hungry!" Dig deeper, why are you hungry and what does your hunger call you to do?

- What would shift if I fasted regularly?

- What breakthrough am I believing for right now—and how can fasting position me for it?

Closing Thought

Men—you weren't made to run from discomfort. You were made to weaponize it.

Fasting isn't a spiritual show—it's a sacred weapon. It silences the noise. Sharpens the spirit. Trains the will. And positions you for power.

Pick up the weapon. Starve the flesh. Feed the spirit.

Fast—and fight.

KINGDOM MEN

Chapter 11: Build Brotherhood

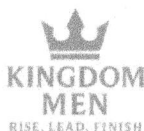

KINGDOM
MEN
RISE, LEAD, FINISH

Key Verse to Memorize:

"Two are better than one... If either of them falls, one can help the other up." — **Ecclesiastes 4:9–10** (NIV)

God's Design: Men Were Made for Brotherhood.

Lone wolves get picked off. Kingdom men run in packs. When men stand shoulder to shoulder, they become a force to be reckoned with.

Brotherhood is not a luxury—it's a Kingdom necessity. God never designed men to walk alone. He designed us for more than casual friendships—He designed us for covenant-level brotherhood. Brotherhood is deeper, stronger, and more dangerous than friendship.

Brotherhood isn't optional for men of God—it's essential. Every man needs brothers who will challenge him, cover him, and call him higher. Men fall when they isolate. But they rise when they link arms, share strength and stand firm. You weren't made to fight alone. You don't need people to like you. You need brothers who fight for you.

The Problem: Brotherhood can be Hard for Men

If you are like me—brotherhood doesn't come easy. We've been burned. We've trusted men who bailed. We fear being exposed. We fear rejection. We'd rather suffer silently than risk connection. These things make isolation seem very appealing. It seems safer to isolate than it does to face the struggle of brotherhood.

But isolation is not harmless—it's a tactic of the enemy. *"A man who isolates himself seeks his own desire; he rages against all wise judgment."* (**Proverbs 18:1**)

Isolation is where men get ambushed. The enemy hunts lone wolves. A man alone is already vulnerable.

Brotherhood in the Arena

When I was fighting bulls, if a bull got a guy down, I would do everything in my power to jump in the middle of the wreck to get the bulls attention so the guy could get away. I didn't look to the stands for help—it was my responsibility. I was my brothers keeper. I trusted whoever I was fighting with and wanted them to be able to trust me.

That's brotherhood. Every man needs someone who runs toward the fight with him, speaks truth when he wants to hide, and reminds him of who he is when he forgets.

Masculine Truth

Real strength is built in godly brotherhood. Take an inventory of the men who have a voice into your life. What is it about them that challenges you to become more like Jesus? You become like the men you surround yourself with—so choose wisely.

- Accountability isn't weakness. Confession isn't failure.

- The man who refuses accountability is already in the enemy's crosshairs.

- Isolation isn't masculine—it's suicidal. The devil doesn't need to kill you if he can separate you.

- Strong men confess. They sharpen one another. They cover each other.

A man alone is a man at risk. A man with brothers is a fortress. Brotherhood is how men sharpen one another to lead and last.

Biblical Anchor: Brotherhood in Scripture

The Bible is filled with examples of covenant brotherhood:

- **David & Jonathan** — Their souls were knit together in covenant (**1 Samuel 18:1**).

- **David's Mighty Men** — They fought beside him, bled with him, and stood their ground (**2 Samuel 23:10**).

- **Shadrach, Meshach, and Abednego** — They faced the fire together and said, *"We will not bow."* (**Daniel 3:18**)

- **Nehemiah's Wall** — Over and over the text reads, *"Next to him... next to him..."* (**Nehemiah 3**). Brotherhood built the wall.

Brotherhood in Scripture is never casual. It's covenant. It's alignment. It's spiritual warfare together. This is the kind of brotherhood that reminds you of your assignment and fights for your future.

The Solution: Jesus as the example-Building Brotherhood

Brotherhood doesn't just happen—it must be built. It takes intentionality, humility, and commitment. Jesus modeled this perfectly. As He walked through life on mission, He gathered men around Him. Men with vision attract other men who are hungry for something more—men who are searching for meaning beyond what they're currently experiencing.

Jesus recognized that hunger in the men He called to follow Him. And those men saw something in Jesus—Messiah, Son of God, the answer they had been looking for.

If you've believed in Jesus for salvation, then you're saved. You're a disciple. And as a disciple, you're also an ambassador of Christ. That means you carry the answer the men around you need—because Jesus is still the answer all men are looking for.

If you want to build strong, lasting brotherhood, live for Jesus. Not just with your words, but with your whole life. He should be evident in your actions, your finances, your emotions, and your health. If you want Kingdom brothers, expand your vision and support other men in expanding and walking out their vision. When the men around you look at your life, can they see Jesus—or just you? Do they see a man on mission who, like Jesus, will expose them to their true God given Identity and calling?

That's the difference between surface-level friendship and Kingdom brotherhood.

Coach's Corner: Four Essentials for Brotherhood

- **Intentionality** — Brotherhood won't build itself. It doesn't happen by accident.

- **Humility** — You have to be willing to open up.

- **Accountability** — Without truth, there's no growth.

- **Commitment** — Show up, even when it's messy.

Ask yourself:

- Who really knows me?

- Who have I invited into my battles?

- Who do I trust to call me out?

Jesus had twelve. David had thirty. Paul had Barnabas and Timothy. You are not the exception. You need brothers too. Who do you have?

Brotherhood: Quality, not Quantity

More doesn't always mean better.

As Gideon grows into his God-given identity as a *mighty man of valor*, we see a powerful lesson in the kind of men God calls us to walk with. **Judges 7:1–7** shows us that the strength of a brotherhood isn't found in numbers—but in the character of the men beside you.

At first, Gideon is surrounded by thousands. Outwardly, it looks like a strong army. But God isn't impressed by numbers. He's after quality. So He begins to separate the courageous from the compromised.

First, He removes 22,000 men who were "fearful and afraid." That's the first test: fear disqualifies a man from the front lines.

Next, God tests them again—this time at the water. Those who dropped to their knees, bowing their faces to the stream and losing sight of their surroundings in pursuit of comfort, were disqualified. They were consumed with satisfying the flesh rather than staying alert.

But 300 men passed the test. They stayed watchful, bringing the water to their mouths while keeping their eyes up. They didn't let thirst distract them from the mission. They were courageous, disciplined, and alert—men God could trust to stand in battle.

You may be surrounded by crowds, but many are still ruled by fear and given over to the flesh.

We are surrounded by men who are the same as the "22,000" that surrounded Gideon. These are not the men you want to link arms with as brothers. Rather, these are the men who need you and your brothers to help them submit to Jesus, realize that they too are sons of God and must rise, lead, and finish all that God has for them.
Ask God to surround you with brothers who are filled with His Spirit—men who are strong, courageous, self-controlled, and focused on the mission. These are the men who won't bow to comfort or shrink back in fear. These are the brothers who will help you advance the Kingdom.

You don't need a crowd. You need godly, courageous, disciplined men. Masculinity cannot be isolated. Every man needs one or two brothers he connects with regularly—men he can be honest with, without posturing or pretending. Real brotherhood involves more than casual conversation; it's rooted in Scripture, confession, prayer, and challenge. It means covering each other's blind spots, protecting each other's marriages, and speaking up before sin has the chance to destroy. It's having someone who holds the line when you're ready to quit—and being that man in return.

This is critical, it's Kingdom strategy.

Qualities of a Kingdom Brotherhood

The kind of brotherhood God builds doesn't happen by accident—you don't stumble into it. You build it with time, trust, and truth. It's made up of men who are Spirit-led, not driven by the flesh. Men who build their bond on truth—not just shared hobbies. It's rooted in vulnerability, not bravado. Marked by real prayer, not empty platitudes. And it's focused on Kingdom purpose— not personal comfort. This is exactly what we see in the life of Gideon. Surrounded at first by thousands, God stripped away the fearful and the ones who let their flesh get in the way of their mission—22,000 men who couldn't carry the weight of advancing the Kingdom. In the end, He left Gideon with 300 men—warriors who were alert, disciplined, and fully surrendered. These are the kind of brothers worth building with.

Core Ideas

- Brotherhood must be intentional, not accidental.

- You become like the men you walk with.

- Isolation is where the enemy does his best work.

- Brotherhood isn't about finding perfect men—it's about becoming stronger men together.

- Brotherhood requires **truth** and **trust.**

- Strong men confess, challenge, and encourage one another.

Questions

- Who is (or isn't) sharpening me?

- Who am I sharpening and who have I failed to sharpen?

- Am I hiding, coasting, or building real brotherhood?

- What fears or pride keep me from inviting others in?

- When was the last time another man challenged my thinking?

- What lies have I believed about asking for help?

- Am I walking alone—or locking arms with brothers?

Call to Action: Build Your Three

Write down the names of three men you trust (or could trust). Pray and ask God who your masculine brothers should be. Reach out to one of them this week and set a time to talk.

Even if it feels awkward. Even if you don't know where to start. Ask real questions. Share real answers. Pray together. Start forming the foundation of brotherhood. Don't wait for it—build it.

Challenge: Weekly Check-In

Choose one man and commit to a weekly check-in. Ask each other three questions:

- How's your heart?

- What are you battling?

- What truth are you standing on?

Make it consistent. Fight together.

Journal Prompts

- Where have I settled for shallow friendships?

- What step can I take this week to forge real brotherhood?

- What do I fear about letting men in?

- What kind of brother do I need to be for others?

- Am I walking alone—or locking arms?

Closing Thought

Men who isolate die slow deaths—emotionally, spiritually, and sometimes physically. But men who link arms together? They become unshakable.

You weren't made to fight alone. You were made for brotherhood. **Link arms. Share strength. Stand firm. Build Brotherhood.**

KINGDOM MEN

Chapter 12: Finish the Race

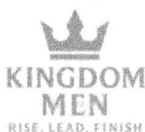

KINGDOM
MEN
RISE, LEAD, FINISH

Key Verses to Memorize:

"I have fought the good fight, I have finished the race, I have kept the faith." — **2 Timothy 4:7**

"...let us lay aside every weight, and the sin which so easily ensnares us, and let us run with endurance the race that is set before us." — **Hebrews 12:1**

Design: God Built Men to Finish

Starting is easy. Finishing strong takes grit. Every man starts with energy. Few finish.

We live in a culture obsessed with hype, momentum, and big starts. But God doesn't crown the man who begins well—He honors the man who finishes well. The man who stays faithful. The man who walks in obedience when it's boring, hard, or lonely.

Paul's final words weren't about his achievements. They were about his endurance:

- "I fought."

- "I finished."
-
- "I kept the faith."

That's the cry of a Kingdom man. Your legacy isn't built on what you begin—it's built on what you bring to completion.

This final chapter is a charge to stay the course—to live and die with nothing left on the table.

Problem: The Danger of Quitting Early

In 2006, I competed in the Dickies National Championship Freestyle Bullfights alongside the PBR in Tulsa, Oklahoma. On the first night, I drew a young bull who was sure enough hot and wanted to fight. He had just enough kick to let me step around him pretty well. The next night I drew a big ole, black, flat-horned bull who had plenty of experience in the fighting arena. Here's what most people don't realize: older bulls learn your "tells." They slow down, wait for you to commit, then ratchet it up a notch and beat you to where you are going. He was that kind of bull.

Before the fight, I was back in the locker room getting taped up. Rex Dunn was kind enough to let me know that the bull I had that night was blind in his left eye. As I went through the fight in my mind, my strategy was to fake to his good eye so he could see me, then I'd step through to his blind side and disappear in hopes of gaining enough time and distance to set the bull up again and keep bringing the fight to him.

Remember, you can throw a fake on a young bull and they'll bite every time. You may be able to throw a fake and step through a handful of times on the same bull, but each time that bull is going to slow up a bit, and then before you know it, you fake one way, go the other and he's there waiting to scoop you up and muck you down. I gave a nod for the gate and the bull came out hot and on the hunt. I squared up, drew him to the right, threw my fake and stepped through then made the rounds with him. At first, it worked, but about 25 seconds into the fight he adjusted. He waited. I hesitated. It was at that point I lost the fight in my mind. I no longer believed I could beat this bull because I didn't think I could get around him. Right at the whistle, he lined me out and hooked me. Technically the fight was over, but, I should have got up and took it to him to make one last round just so I could end on my terms rather than his. I didn't. Not getting back up and stepping to him is the only regret of my 16 years in the arena—not that I lost, but that I didn't finish strong.

Dr. Edwin Louis Cole said, "Winners are not those who never fail, but those who never quit." I failed and quit…and still regret it.

That's how many men live. They start bold but lose their fight. They hesitate. They let regret creep in because they fail to finish on God's terms. If that's you, I need you to get up. Your family needs you to get up. There are people counting on you. You need to make the decision to get up and step back into the fight.

Masculine Truth

Men don't drift to the finish line—they decide their way there. Masculinity decides to get back up even after getting worked over in the arena. Finishing strong isn't glamorous, in fact, it looks a lot like getting stomped on and mauled by obstacles in life, then you get up, spit the dirt and blood out of your teeth and step back to the bull.

- You don't need to be the most talented—you need to consistently get back up and learn.

- Finishing is about daily decisions.

- A finisher doesn't burn out, bow out, or back down.

- He lives faithful to his calling, his wife, his children, and God.

A finisher dies empty of regret because he poured everything out. This means letting go of failure and regret and asking Holy Spirit to heal you so you can confidently move forward.

Injured in the Fight

Cowboys compete with injuries. It's just part of the job. I was fighting bulls at a PBR Cody Custer was putting on in Missoula, Montana when I took a horn under my vest and broke two ribs. I still had 25 bulls left plus the short round. I gritted my teeth, fought through the pain, and finished my job. That wasn't the only time—broken ribs, dislocated shoulders, separated sternums—there were many injuries that challenged me to quit, I fought through it.

Every event I started, I finished. Every event but one. Because every man has a breaking point. And that's where grace is found.

Masculinity calls men to finish what they start, that's at the heart of who we are. Masculinity challenges a man to own his responsibility, not make excuses. Men show up. Men finish.

Biblical Anchor: Jesus the Finisher

- Noah spent 100+ years building an ark. He finished.

- Paul endured shipwrecks, stoning, and prisons—and still finished his race.

At the end of his life, Paul doesn't boast about how many churches he planted or how many miracles he saw.

He simply says:

"I have fought the good fight."
"I have finished the race."
"I have kept the faith."

And Jesus? He didn't just die. He finished. His final words on the cross weren't, *"I did my best"*—they were: "It is finished." (**John 19:30**) He completed His assignment. He endured the cross. He fulfilled prophecy. He left nothing undone.

A Kingdom man follows His example. He doesn't just start strong— he finishes strong.

Solution: 3 Keys to Finishing the Race

1. Stay Focused on the Vision
"Fix your eyes on Jesus, the author and finisher of your faith..." (**Hebrews 12:2**) Vision leaks. You need daily reminders. Write your Vision and your "why" where you can see it. Read it. Speak it. Declare it.

2. Refuse to Run Alone
"Run in such a way... not without aim." (**1 Corinthians 9:26**) Isolated men run away from challenges. Brotherhood keeps you accountable, encouraged, and corrected. Brothers encourage you to run toward the challenges that stand in your way and threaten to keep you from walking in your God-given identity.

3. Train with Discipline

"Everyone who competes in the games goes into strict training." (**1 Corinthians 9:25**) Discipline is the bridge between desire and destiny. You must discipline your mind to think like Jesus so you can be and do like Jesus. Train your body, mind, and spirit. Show up even when motivation is gone.

Coach's Corner

I was teaching a fighting school when one of my students got mucked out. It wasn't anything too serious, but it rattled him enough that he panicked, bailed over the fence, and ran out of the arena.

I walked over to him and asked, "Why did you run?"

He said, "Because I couldn't breathe."

I told him, "The air on this side of the fence is the same as the air on that side. What made you run wasn't a lack of oxygen—it was fear. Fear convinced you that you had to escape. But if you keep listening to fear, you'll always run from the very thing that's meant to shape you. The only way forward is to get back in the arena, face it, and fight again."

You've fought too many battles to let fear deceive you into jumping the fence in an effort to escape the pressure God can use to refine you.

Ask yourself:

- Where have I run in fear when I needed to stay and fight?

- What arena has God called me to fight in?

- What am I still called to build, protect, or complete?

- What excuses do I need to kill to finish strong?

Legacy isn't what you say—it's what remains when you are gone.

Core Truths

- Good intentions don't leave a godly legacy—faithful actions do.

- A strong start means little if you don't finish.

- Consistency builds impact. Obedience builds legacy.

- Finishers live with eternity in mind.

Questions for Reflection

- Where have I stopped short in my calling or leadership?

- Am I building toward legacy—or coasting in comfort?

- What daily habits are shaping my finish line?

- Who's watching how I run—and what are they learning?

- What areas of my life are unfinished—and why?

- What would it look like to end well—spiritually, physically, relationally, emotionally, and financially?

- What's the legacy I want to leave—and am I living like it matters?

Action Steps

- **Identify Three Areas to Finish Strong**

within each of the 5 listed areas below, identify 3 things you know you need to finish strong.

- Spiritual health—*examples: leading myself/family in reading the Word, Prayer, Corporate worship.*

- Physical health—*examples: healthy diet, exercise, rest.*

- Relational health- *example building brotherhood, restoring broken relationships, stewarding my family.*

- Emotional health—*examples: Receive and give forgiveness, walk free of fear and anxiety.*

- Financial health—*examples: lifestyle of generosity, tithing, investing.*

- **Name the Finish Line**
  Define what "finishing strong" looks like in those areas.

- **Declare War on Distraction**
  Remove things that pull you away from the goal.

- **Commit to Brotherhood**
  Share your finish line with a brother who will hold you accountable.

- **Make a Finish Line Covenant**
  Write this in your journal and declare it out loud:
  "I am a Kingdom man.
  I finish my race. I will keep the faith.
  I walk with endurance. I do not quit when it's hard.
  I rely on His strength, not mine.
  I am faithful in season and out.
  I will finish well—by His grace."

Say it out loud every day this week before your feet hit the floor.

Then take action like a man on a mission.

Journal Prompt

- If I continue on this path, what will my legacy be?

- What am I proud to have finished?

- What have I avoided finishing—and why?

- What will I recommit to finishing today?

You were built to finish.

Run hard. End well. Leave a legacy worth following.

Final Word: When You Break

Let's revisit the fighting event I started and didn't finish. A bull pitched me in the air and when I came down, I landed on my back, breaking it. I could stand, but had no lateral movement and could hardly walk. That was the only event I started and didn't finish. This was my breaking point.

In life, we all have one. You've had yours. I've had mine. And when it comes, this is the truth:

- Repentance is the path to restoration.

- You are not disqualified.

- God has not changed His mind about you (**Romans 11:29**).

Men may try to disqualify you. Many times they will use scripture to do it—but God has the final word. He is with you when you finish strong, and He is with you when you fail miserably. Either
way, He still has plans for you. He's not done with you. Don't quit.

There is hope. Get back up. Dust yourself off. Discover your identity, gain God's vision and fulfill your calling. Get back in the fight!

The Greatest Problem Every Man Faces

This book is built on a *problem/solution* framework using a strategic approach to increasing satisfaction in life. The method is simple: **parts, practices, outcome**. If a man wants to grow in any area, he must be able to identify the real problem, understand what fuels it, recognize the behaviors that flow from it, see the outcome it produces.

With that said, it would be impossible to talk about life, strength, or purpose without addressing the biggest problem every man faces:

Separation From God

Scripture pulls no punches on this.
Romans 3:23, Romans 5:12, Ephesians 2:3, and 1 Corinthians 15:22 make it clear: **every man is born into sin**, and sin separates us from a holy God.

The cost of that sin is death (Romans 6:23; 5:6–8).
That's the problem—and it's a debt no man can pay on his own. The payment required is a perfect sacrifice, and none of us qualify.
We've all been marked by sin.

But God didn't leave us there.
In His mercy and strength, He stepped into our world, took on flesh, and went to the cross to pay the debt we couldn't. In the ultimate act of love and courage, *"while we were still sinners, Christ died for us."*

Jesus traded His life for ours.
He opened the door to eternal life—and eternal life isn't something that begins after you die. **It begins now. It's meant to be lived on earth with the same power and presence that exists in heaven.**

The Free Gift of Salvation

You can't earn this gift. You can't prove yourself worthy of it.
It is given freely to every man who calls on the name of Jesus.

If you've never received this gift—and you want to—this is your moment.

Romans 10:9–10 lays it out clearly:
"If you confess with your mouth that Jesus is Lord and believe in your heart that God raised Him from the dead, you will be saved."

If you're ready, pray this:

Prayer of Salvation

Father, I am a sinner. Your Word says my sin separates me from You, and that the wages of sin is death.
I deserve that penalty and in your great love, you took that penalty for me when you sent Jesus to die in my place.
Jesus, I believe You are Lord and that You rose from the dead, conquering death and the grave.
You have given that victory to me.
From this day forward, teach me to live for You. Show me who You are and who You created me to be.
Thank You. Amen.

Jesus said, *"I am the Way, the Truth, and the Life. No one comes to the Father except through Me."*

He is the solution to our separation problem.
He restores what sin destroyed.
He reconnects us to the Father so we never have to live disconnected again.

Epilogue:

Kingdom Men Advance

What's next? You've walked through a battle plan. You've been called up higher. Now, it's time to live it out.

Kingdom men *advance*. They take ground for God's Kingdom, wherever they go. They are called to become like Jesus. To do this, you'll need men around you to lead you, walk with you and support you. It would also be wise to find a good mentor and or coach. I'd love to help you along the way. I offer individual and group coaching, retreats and accountability and have more books coming.
Please reach out at Kingdommencoaching.com and let me know how I can best serve you.

ABOUT THE AUTHOR

Dusty Lapp is a husband, father, minister, mentor, coach, and teacher. In 2006 he was Commissioned a Minister to Men by Faithful Men Ministries. His life's work has been shaped by a unique blend of grit, faith, and relentless pursuit of growth.

Dusty holds a Master's degree in Life Coaching and Mentorship and an undergraduate degree in Christian Management and Leadership. He is a John Maxwell Certified Coach and Trainer, a Certified Couple and Core Communication Instructor, Nutritional Therapy Practitioner, Precision Nutrition Level 2 Master Health Coach, and a National Board Certified Health and Wellness Coach.

Dusty spent **16 years fighting bulls in the PBR and PRCA**. The arena taught him lessons about people, pressure, and identity that continue to shape the way he leads, coaches and mentors today.

For more than two decades, Dusty's mission is to Connect with Leaders, Grow their Influence, Expand their Impact, and Support them to lead others.

Dusty has served on multiple boards, including **Riding High Ministries** (2013–2019), where he later became Board Chair (2019–2021), and the **Nutritional Therapy Association** (2018–2019). His ministry work has taken him to prisons, churches, and communities across the U.S., Europe, and Africa carrying a message of hope and a bold call for men to rise up, embrace true masculinity, and lead with courage.

In addition to ministry, Dusty has built and operated multiple businesses across various industries, blending practical leadership with Kingdom principles. His life and work are marked by a single focus: walk as son and help men discover their God given identity, gain vision and fulfill their calling—Romans 8:19.

www.ingramcontent.com/pod-product-compliance
Lightning Source LLC
Chambersburg PA
CBHW052136270326
41930CB00012B/2912